T0047163

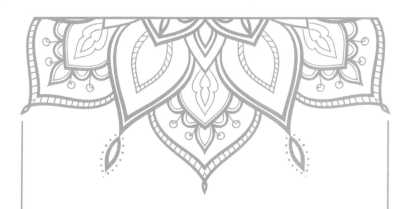

MY POCKET
GUIDE
~ TO ~
STRETCHING

ANYTIME STRETCHES FOR FLEXIBILITY,
STRENGTH, AND FULL-BODY WELLNESS

K. ALEISHA FETTERS, CSCS

ADAMS MEDIA
NEW YORK   LONDON   TORONTO   SYDNEY   NEW DELHI

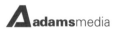

Adams Media
An Imprint of Simon & Schuster, Inc.
100 Technology Center Drive
Stoughton, Massachusetts 02072

First Adams Media trade paperback edition March 2022

ADAMS MEDIA and colophon are trademarks of Simon & Schuster.

For information about special discounts for bulk purchases, please contact Simon & Schuster Special Sales at 1-866-506-1949 or business@simonandschuster.com.

The Simon & Schuster Speakers Bureau can bring authors to your live event. For more information or to book an event contact the Simon & Schuster Speakers Bureau at 1-866-248-3049 or visit our website at www.simonspeakers.com.

Interior design by Michelle Kelly
Interior images by Eric Andrews; © 123RF/Viktory

Manufactured in China

10 9 8 7 6 5 4 3 2 1

Library of Congress Cataloging-in-Publication Data has been applied for.

ISBN 978-1-5072-1795-5
ISBN 978-1-5072-1796-2 (ebook)

CONTENTS

PART 3: SEQUENCES FOR EVERY STRETCHING NEED / 133

INTRODUCTION

Looking for an easy, portable collection of stretches you can do whenever and wherever? Look no further. Whether you're new to stretching or you've been practicing for years, *My Pocket Guide to Stretching* will help you loosen, relax, and elongate your muscles throughout the day. The moves, twists, and bends you'll find in this guide will help you feel more balanced, centered, and refreshed in minutes. Stressed? Tight shoulders? Back pain? Can't sleep? There's a stretch—and even a full sequence of stretches—for that.

You've no doubt heard about the benefits of stretching before exercising. By readying your body for a greater range of motion during exercise, you're preparing yourself for a more effective exercise session and a lower chance of injury. But the benefits of stretching go far beyond productive exercise. Regular stretching can help you relieve tension and pain, open and strengthen your body, quiet and focus your mind, relieve tension, increase your body awareness, and vastly improve the quality of your life. By practicing stretches, you activate your body's reset button. When day-to-day life causes wear and tear on your body, allow stretching to be your solution. Sitting for long periods of time shortens the muscles in the front of your hips, limiting your flexibility and worsening your posture. Looking down at your phone tightens your neck and shoulder muscles. Even healthy activities such as lifting weights can cause muscle imbalances, aches, and pains when done incorrectly. Only by stretching your body from head to toe can you switch back to your musculoskeletal system's default, and ideal, setting.

My Pocket Guide to Stretching also teaches you how to use stretching to not just benefit your body, but to also care for your emotional and mental health. You'll complete specific stretches for stress and anxiety relief, lowering blood pressure, getting better sleep, and more. You'll learn to incorporate mindfulness into your stretching practice, focusing on the present moment and letting go of all worries as you stretch.

The stretches in this book will help you become more flexible, calm, and restored—in body and mind. Let's get started.

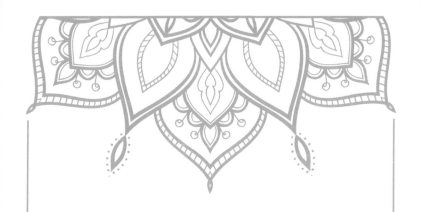

PART 1

HOW TO STRETCH FOR THE BEST RESULTS

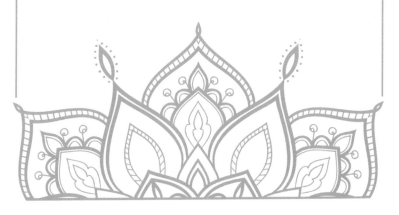

Before you attempt stretching, it's important to have a full understanding of what exactly stretching is, how it works, and why it's so important for your health. In this part, you'll learn all of that, as well as the importance of knowing your limits, why you shouldn't overstretch, and how to avoid injury while stretching. You'll become familiar with the science behind stretching, and how it benefits not only your body but also your mind.

THE BENEFITS OF STRETCHING

Most people start stretching because they want one very specific thing: flexibility. That's all well and good. After all, a consistent stretching practice is one of the most beneficial (not to mention easiest) ways to improve your muscle flexibility and even your joint mobility. Your *flexibility* is the extent to which you can stretch your muscles. Your mobility is how easily your joints move through their full and healthy range of motion. In this book, some stretches will focus on lengthening muscles such as the glutes, quads, and back muscles, while others will increase mobility in joints like the shoulders, hips, and wrists.

But saying that stretching is all about flexibility or mobility sells stretching short. Here, you'll learn some of the other important benefits of having a regular stretching habit.

Stretching Aligns Your Posture

Muscle tightness and joint restrictions are synonymous with poor posture. Fortunately, the tightness and restrictions caused by poor posture can be alleviated by proper stretching exercises.

Take your hip joint, for example. In your hip joint, you've got your pelvis and your femur (thigh bone) that connects to it. On one side of the joint, you've got all your hip flexors, which bend the joint. This includes your quadriceps (quads), iliopsoas, and other little muscles you may not know about. On the other side of the joint are your gluteal muscles (glutes) and hamstrings.

When your hip flexors are tight (as is common with runners, cyclists, and anyone who sits a lot), they pull the front of your pelvis down toward your femur. This is called an anterior pelvic tilt. There's an arch in your lower back, your glutes are pushed out behind you, and your hamstrings feel extremely tight. That's because when your pelvis tilts down in the front, your glutes tilt up in the back—constantly pulling your hamstrings tight like a rubber band. Stretching and elongating your hip flexors can actually help your hamstrings *feel* like they're loosening up.

Examples of muscle tightness abound in the body. Just look to any joint (your neck, shoulders, back, elbows, wrists, knees, ankles), and you'll find opposing muscles in a tug of war...when what you really want are smooth-flowing, equally pulling-and-tugging motions.

Stretching helps to ever-so-gently restore that relationship. As a result, your joints sit in their proper place and move how they are meant to move. And when the hundreds of bones in your body can move the right way, your body also moves better and works more efficiently.

Stretching Lowers Your Risk of Aches, Pains, and Injury

Using the hip joint as another example, let's think about what else happens when your pelvis tilts and pulls your hamstrings tight. First, you throw off your body's center of gravity and move it *outside* of your body. As your pelvis tilts forward in the front and backward in the back, and your lower back arches, your center of gravity moves to where your lower back used to be—right in that little divot. This puts extra stress, or weight, into those muscles, making them work overtime and causing pain and tightness.

Meanwhile, with the extra stress on your posture, you're not able to take advantage of your glutes' or hamstrings' full strength. As a result, your running pace might stall, or you might get winded taking the stairs. In the worst-case scenario, as other muscles work to pick up the slack and help your hips continue to move, you might experience an injury.

Stretching helps to fortify not just your muscles but also your tendons, ligaments, and even cartilage, thus helping to avoid injuries. Tendons connect muscles to bones, and ligaments connect bones to other bones. By moving your joints through their full range of motion, you help deliver nutrient-rich blood to your tendons and ligaments, and also warm them, which improves their elasticity. Stretching helps reduce the risk of strains and sprains as well as overuse issues like having runner's knee or tennis elbow.

Stretching Boosts Your Exercise Warm-Up and Recovery

Getting the blood (and all of its oxygen and other nutrients) flowing is especially important before and after any physical activity, regardless of whether you're jogging, cycling, lifting weights, or climbing.

As you prepare your body for exercise, a gentle stretching session takes your joints through their full range of motion, increases blood flow to your muscles and connective tissues, and literally raises the body's core temperature. A stretching session also causes your muscles to accumulate calcium ions. Your muscles use these molecules to contract, work their best, and help you achieve your fitness goals.

Many times at the end of workouts, exercised muscles—the ones that have been contracting hard throughout your sweat session—can feel tight and almost "locked" in a contracted position. You can use stretching to relax worked muscles back to their proper resting length and position. Stretching can also be a gentle way to lower your heart rate and blood pressure after a workout, as well as an opportunity to check in with your body. Use your post-workout stretch routines to get a feel for how your body has responded to your workout and identify any stiffness or pain in your muscle groups or joints that might need stretching or more recovery time before your next workout.

Stretching Reduces Your Stress Levels

People tend to carry stress in their muscles, and stretching is a great tool to release that muscular tension—and even manage emotional and mental stress.

When you stretch, your body's levels of mood-regulating signaling chemicals, called neurotransmitters, increase. Two of the most researched chemicals include dopamine and serotonin. Both are linked with feelings of relaxation and pleasure in the brain. Meanwhile, a large portion of your body's serotonin receptors are actually in your gastrointestinal system. Research has also shown that serotonin promotes healthy gut function. In fact, selective serotonin reuptake inhibitors (SSRIs), medications that work to increase the levels of serotonin in the body, have proven helpful in easing gastrointestinal issues such as irritable bowel syndrome (IBS).

All chemistry aside, stretching is an opportunity to practice mindfulness, which is hugely beneficial for mental and emotional health. By focusing on the present moment, you step away from your worries of the future and ruminations of the past, and are able to effectively manage your stress. To get the greatest mindfulness benefits of stretching, during your sessions, resist the urge to absentmindedly scroll through your newsfeed or think about your to-do list, which will still be there waiting for you when you're done. Breathe slowly and deeply and focus all your attention on what you feel in your body and how your body reacts to subtle changes in position.

Stretching Improves Your Sleep Quality

Among the myriad calming benefits of stretching, a regular stretching practice can also help you sleep better. You'll sleep better if stretching is a part of your daily life—whether you stretch throughout the day or add in a stretching routine before bedtime.

Remember, at the end of the day, your body and muscles carry all of the emotions (and uncomfortable postures) you've experienced throughout the day (read: they're tight). Stretching helps to release this tension, get your muscles to their ideal resting length, and realign your spine and joints. As a result, you may fall asleep faster, sleep more soundly, and even wake up with fewer aches.

Stretching Strengthens Your Muscles

Tight muscles are weak muscles. For example, if you're hunched over a phone all day with rounded shoulders and tight back muscles, your upper back is, without question, weakened. The same goes for your glutes, which sit inactive all day if you work at a desk.

While stretching is no substitute for regular resistance exercise, it can help you maximize your muscle strength. In fact, a *Medicine & Science in Sports & Exercise* study reported that people who stretched their legs for forty minutes a few times a week significantly improved their lower-body strength—without doing any other exercise. They also improved their muscular endurance and the height and length of their jumps.

HOW DOES STRETCHING WORK?

Though scientists are continuing to research stretching and its many effects on the body, its positive results are certain. Here's a closer look at the anatomy and physiology of stretching.

Stretching Literally Stretches Your Muscles

Your muscles and connective tissues are all a certain length; they connect from one part of a bone to one part of another bone. So, by moving your bones—spine, arms, hips, legs—to their end ranges of motion, you effectively increase the distance between those two points, causing the muscles to stretch to their natural "resting length."

Stretching Boosts Blood Flow

Everything in your body needs blood—and the nutrients, like oxygen, it carries. Your cardiovascular system is always pumping and moving this life force throughout your body, but it does its best job when you're active and moving. Case in point: At rest, your joints get very little blood flow. That's why exercise physiologists often call joints, and especially cartilage (the padding at the end of your bones) "blood poor." Dynamic stretching—moving your joints gently—actively forces blood and nutrients into those thirsty tissues.

Stretching Trains Your Nervous System

Your autonomic (unconscious) nervous system plays an important role in your body's flexibility and mobility. Within each of your muscles, you have stretch-sensors called muscle spindles. Whenever you stretch a muscle, these sensors gauge how far you're lengthening it and how quickly you're doing so. If you're stretching deeper or your movements are faster than usual, your muscle spindles send an alert signal to your brain to make your muscle contract. After all, the muscle spindles' mission is to protect your muscles from stretching too far or tearing.

But remember, your body raises the alarm if you stretch your muscles far beyond their normal length. So, by gently and consistently stretching, you train your muscle spindles. They learn to let you use your natural full range of motion to maybe touch your toes, as opposed to contracting muscles when you get to your knees. In other words, stretching helps you teach your nervous system to let you move in ways you couldn't before.

STATIC VERSUS DYNAMIC STRETCHING

Bend down and try to touch your toes and remain in this position for at least thirty seconds. If you can, try this simple stretch for a minute or two. This stretch is an example of static stretching. Now, stand with your feet together (and hold on to something for balance). Keeping one knee straight, or as straight as you can, gently swing that leg behind and then in front of your body, back-and-forth, again and again. This is dynamic stretching.

If you tried both of these stretches, you undoubtedly felt both of them in one main place: your hamstrings. After all, both stretches moved your hip joint through its full range of motion and stretched, or pulled, your hamstrings to their full resting length.

So why would you do one type of stretching instead of the other? The answer comes down to what you want to get out of any one stretch session.

Static Stretching

Traditional bend-and-hold stretches—like the ones you probably did back in your gym class days when you would sit on the floor and try to touch your toes—pull your muscles hard, which is great for increasing muscle flexibility.

But bend-and-hold stretches can work to your disadvantage right before a workout. After all, your muscles are elastic, like rubber bands. And if you stretch a rubber band out as hard as possible and then try to slingshot it, it probably won't go very far. The same holds true for your muscles before exercise, with long, static stretches decreasing your muscles' elastic qualities and, thus, their ability to generate maximal force. Studies show that holding static stretches for more than thirty seconds immediately before a workout reduces your muscles' strength and power. In fact, the American College of Sports Medicine has specifically advised against static stretching before workouts and competitions.

That said, static stretches are great after exercising when you're trying to bring your heart rate down and relax your body. Spend at least five minutes on static stretches after each workout, immediately following a light aerobic cooldown like walking.

For even greater benefits, try doing static stretches throughout the day whenever the urge strikes. After all, one of the pros of static stretches is that they're simple and accessible. For example, when you're in the office, bending down to touch your toes might be easier to pull off (and will likely result in fewer stares!) than swinging your leg back-and-forth. Similarly, because you don't have to move around, static stretches are easy to do in bed as part of your going-to-sleep or waking-up routine.

Dynamic Stretching

By and large, dynamic stretches don't pull your muscles quite as tight as static moves do. Because dynamic stretches are gentler on your muscles, they won't impede your workout performance the way pre-run or pre-lifting static stretches can. Research shows, rather, that dynamic stretches can majorly benefit your workouts and athletic performance.

That's because dynamic stretches don't just work your muscle flexibility—they also optimize your joint mobility. With each move, you take one or more joints through their full range of motion, which not only prepares your joints, cartilage, tendons, and ligaments for the workout ahead; it also helps shuttle blood and oxygen to all of your working tissues.

Dynamic stretching even causes your muscles to accumulate calcium ions. Calcium ions are molecules that help your muscles contract and work their best. So by preloading your muscles with calcium ions through dynamic movements, you "prime the pump," so to speak.

Consider dynamic stretches a staple of your warm-up routine. Ideally, you should spend a good five to ten minutes moving and stretching before your workouts. The key is to focus on joints and movement patterns that mimic the exercise you're about to do. For instance, if you're going to go for a run, you'll want to do some lunges with standing reaches and leg swings (see Part 2). If you're going to do some bench and shoulder presses, try Wall Slides (see Part 2) for your dynamic stretch.

WHEN AND HOW OFTEN SHOULD YOU STRETCH?

As you just read, stretching before and after exercise is important for different reasons. But stretching sessions don't have to coincide with your workout time. It's rare that stretching too much would cause any issues—especially if you stretch properly and don't push yourself to the point of pain.

For instance, Harvard Medical School recommends that people stretch all of their muscles and tendons, from head to toes, at least two to three times per week. And, a *Journal of Strength and Conditioning Research* study of people ages eighteen to forty-six found that stretching a total of six times per week delivers the best results for the effort. The study found that in order to achieve six stretch sessions per week, the same results are obtained by stretching multiple times each day. The researchers also found that, while more is generally better when it comes to stretching, people who spent between three and seventeen total minutes per week stretching enjoyed major flexibility and mobility benefits.

When trying to figure out the best stretching schedule for you, simply listen to your body. It'll tell you when your shoulders are feeling knotted up or your calves are tight. Respond, in kind, with a few minutes of stretching. By incorporating short stretching sessions into your day, you're more likely to catch tension and tightness before they turn into a full-blown migraine or back spasm. Also, when you deliberately tune in to your body more often, you're more likely to hold yourself accountable to your stretching goals.

Try making stretching the very first thing you do in the morning. Start your day with several stretches to wake up your body and stretch the muscles that have been lying dormant for (hopefully) seven to nine hours. Throughout the day, get away from your desk and stretch—or do stretches right at your desk. You'll find plenty of stretches in this guide that are desk-friendly. Before bed, tune in to how you're feeling and loosen up any muscles or joints that feel tight. You'll calm your body and will be able to drift off sooner. (Turn to Part 3 for a nighttime stretch routine you can do right in bed.)

DON'T OVERSTRETCH!

The phrase "no pain, no gain" doesn't hold true when it comes to stretching. When you stretch too hard, you risk harming your muscles and connective tissues, and causing a strain, which happens when a muscle or tendon stretches too far. You also risk causing a sprain, which is when your ligaments stretch too far. With either straining and spraining, you risk tearing body tissue.

The difference between stretching and damaging tissue lies in the intensity of the stretch. Pain is your body's way of alerting you that something is wrong, and pain during stretching usually means that you're overstretching. Pay attention, and do whatever you need to do to end the pain, like not trying to reach as far during a stretch and instead letting your body ease into it. It doesn't matter if you can't clasp your hands behind your back right now. Do what you can, and do it comfortably. With consistent practice, you'll be able to gradually progress deeper into your stretches, and without pain.

It's also important to mention that bouncing does not help flexibility. People tend to bounce during their stretches to push themselves harder or to make their muscles stretch farther. Think back to elementary school when your gym teacher had you do the butterfly stretch. You sat on the floor, placed the soles of your feet together, and pulled them in close to your body. You were most likely coached to flap your knees up and down in order to become more flexible. This bouncing was actually harmful. Stretching too fast makes your muscles contract and actively fight your stretching attempts. This contraction works in direct opposition of your goals. It limits your ability to stretch your muscles and move through full ranges of motion. More concerningly, it increases your risk of hurting your muscles and connective tissues. Stretching an actively squeezing (contracting) muscle can damage its contractile components, again increasing your risk of strains.

Remember that stretching is not a contest; it's about giving your body what it needs. If you follow this simple principle, you'll be setting yourself up for a lifetime of health benefits.

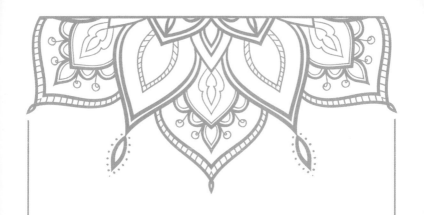

PART 2

STRETCH BY BODY PART

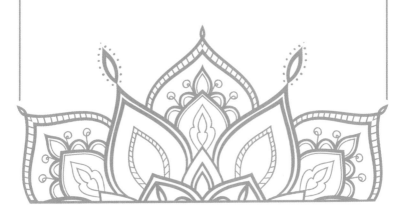

This part contains more than fifty popular stretches that you can turn to again and again in your daily life. Read through the description and look at the figures before doing a stretch to get familiar with the shape and actions of it. Remember to breathe continuously and smoothly while stretching. Don't get discouraged if the stretches seem difficult at first; that's normal. Remember to not push yourself past your limits. With gentle practice, your muscles will become accustomed to the movements, and you'll be able to achieve longer and deeper stretches.

Segmented Chin Square

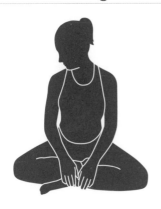 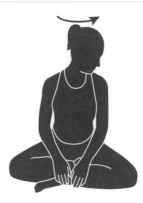

Your neck is made to move in so many directions, but most days, you probably don't make many of these movements. And, like any joint, your neck operates with a use-it-or-lose-it mentality. This dynamic stretch takes advantage of four separate end ranges of motion to help you preserve and even expand mobility. This stretch isn't something you can do while you're on your phone or run through absentmindedly. Focus on moving purposefully. Throughout the entire stretch, keep your shoulder blades pulled gently down and together, which will help brace your shoulders. This will also help you relax your upper trapezius and improve posture.

Benefits
* Relieves tension through the upper traps and sternocleidomas-toid muscles (the side of the neck).
* Maintains and improves healthy range of motion in the neck.
* Helps relax the shoulders down and away from the ears for better posture.
* Calms the mind and relieves stress.

Steps:
1. Sit tall on the floor or in a chair with your shoulders relaxed and hands in your lap.
2. Drop your chin and point it toward one shoulder. Pause.
3. Raise your chin straight up over that shoulder. Pause.
4. Move your chin straight to the side over your other shoulder. Pause.
5. Drop your chin straight down to that shoulder. Pause.
6. Repeat all steps, then switch directions.

To Deepen This Stretch...
* Walk your hands out to your sides on the floor. Stay in this position throughout the entire exercise.
* Let your head drop slightly behind you, aligning your chin over your shoulder blades.

Ear-to-Shoulder

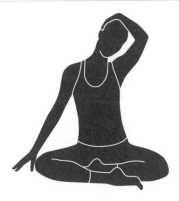

You've probably done this static stretch in some form, most likely while sitting in a desk chair. Doing it with proper form allows you to get an even better release for looser muscles. A common error during this exercise is dropping your gaze to the floor. Keep your face pointed at the wall in front of you. Also, keep your shoulder blades pulled gently down and together to brace and stabilize your shoulders.

Benefits

* Relieves tension through the upper traps and sternocleidomastoid muscles (the side of the neck).
* Maintains and improves healthy range of motion in the neck.
* Helps relax the shoulders down and away from the ears for better posture.
* Eases stress headaches.

Steps:

1. Sit tall on the floor or in a chair with your shoulders down and hands in your lap.
2. Place one hand on the opposite side of your head, above your

ear. Gently and slowly pull your head to draw your ear toward that side's shoulder.

3. Hold, then switch sides.

To Deepen This Stretch...

* Place your free hand on the floor and walk it straight out to your side until you feel the stretch into your shoulder.

* Place the back of your free hand on the middle of your back.

Chin-to-Chest Pull

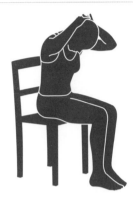

Your spine spends so much of the day rounding forward, so you might be surprised how amazing it feels to actively pull your chin forward to your chest. That's because, with this static stretch, you're not actively putting weight into your back-of-the-neck muscles. Instead, you're lengthening them to their end range of motion, a position you likely don't use when texting. After all, when you're on your phone, you're not trying to look at your navel. But with this stretch, that's exactly what you'll do.

Benefits
* Relieves tension through the upper traps, rhomboids (between the shoulder blades and the spine), and splenius capitis (in the back of the neck).
* Maintains and improves healthy range of motion in the neck.
* Helps relax the shoulders down and away from the ears for better posture.

* Improves form during upper-body exercises like rows and presses.

Steps:
1. Sit tall on the floor or in a chair with the fingers of both hands interlaced behind the base of your head.
2. Gently and slowly pull your hands into your head to round your cervical spine and draw your chin down to your chest.
3. Hold.

To Deepen This Stretch...
 * Gently round the upper part of your thoracic spine between your shoulder blades.
 * As you breathe, imagine trying to inflate the stretched muscles.

Behind-the-Back Lock

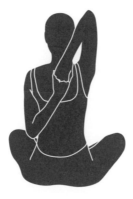

A great test of shoulder mobility—and a great way to train it—this stretch has the ultimate goal of touching (or hooking) your fingers together behind your back, between your shoulder blades. Reaching this end range of motion, though, can be very challenging, so don't push it. Focus on moving only as far as actually feels good. If you end up being able to touch your fingers together, that's great. If not, just keep practicing.

Benefits

* Improves shoulder mobility and function, guarding against common shoulder restrictions.
* Trains the rotator cuff muscles and connective tissues.
* Helps ease the kyphosis (rounded upper spine) that can occur with frequent computer, tablet, and phone use, as well as with aging.
* Improves coordination and proprioception, the sense of the body's positioning and movements.
* Reduces the risk of shoulder injury.

Steps:
1. Extend one arm overhead, then bend your elbow to place your palm on your upper back.
2. Letting your other arm hang straight at your side, bend that elbow to place the back of your hand against your lower back.
3. Moving from your shoulders, slide your hands toward each other. Your top elbow should point toward the ceiling, and your bottom elbow toward the floor.
4. Hold, then switch sides.

To Deepen This Stretch...
* Use each exhale to help you bring your hands closer together.
* If you have trouble holding the position, hold one end of a resistance band in your top hand. Grab the other end with your bottom hand.

Cross-Body Shoulder Stretch

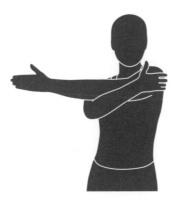

If you want to stretch your deltoid muscles, this static stretch has you covered. It focuses on the posterior, or back, portion of your shoulder muscles to get you in a more upright posture. This stretch also maximizes your shoulder mobility because it moves your shoulder in ways you wouldn't normally move it in your day-to-day life. When doing this exercise, play with the positioning of your working shoulder. This stretch targets slightly different muscle fibers depending on whether you let your shoulder round forward against your chest or if you keep it pulled back and your chest tall.

Benefits
* Relieves tension through the rear (posterior) deltoid, teres minor and major, and supraspinatus in the back of the shoulder.
* Improves shoulder mobility and function, guarding against common shoulder restrictions.
* Helps ease the kyphosis (rounded upper spine) that can occur with frequent computer, tablet, and phone use, as well as with aging.

* Improves form during upper-body exercises such as rows and presses (when done dynamically).

Steps:

1. Reach across your chest with one arm, keeping your elbow straight.
2. Wrap your other arm under it and place your hand on your upper arm.
3. Gently pull your extended arm toward your chest.
4. Hold, then switch sides.

To Deepen This Stretch...

* Place your hand on your forearm, rather than on your upper arm. Keep your stretched arm's elbow straight.
* To make the stretch dynamic, after you pull your arm to your chest, slowly move it away from your chest.

Reverse Shoulder Raise

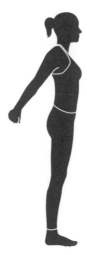

This static stretch focuses on the muscles in front of your shoulder. When stretching, it's important to hit both sides of any joint. This helps reduce the risk of, and eases existing, muscle imbalances. In day-to-day life, the front (anterior) deltoids don't spend much time in a stretched position. Rather, they tend to hang out in a shortened, or contracted, position. Releasing the tension here reduces their pull forward. Keep in mind, though, that because you don't move in this position often, it can feel very intense, challenging, or even impossible at first. If that's the case for you, keep trying daily in order to see results with time and practice.

Benefits

* Relieves tension through the anterior deltoid and pectoralis major in the front of the shoulder.

* Helps ease the kyphosis (rounded upper spine) that can occur with frequent computer, tablet, and phone use, as well as with aging.
* Improves shoulder mobility and function, guarding against common shoulder restrictions.

Steps:

1. Interlace the fingers of both hands behind your back with your arms against the back of your hips.
2. Keeping your spine tall, and not leaning through your lower back, lift your arms toward the ceiling behind you.
3. Hold.

To Deepen This Stretch...

* After interlacing your fingers, rotate your palms toward your hips and then down to the floor. Maintain this position as you raise your arms.

Active Shoulder Roll

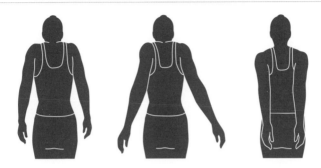

When doing a shoulder roll, you really feel the stretch through both sides of your deltoids as well as through your shoulder blades as you actively work and contract your muscles. To do a shoulder roll properly, it's helpful to think back to the Cross-Body Shoulder Stretch, where you use one shoulder's muscles to move your other shoulder through its full range of motion and stretch its muscles. In the Active Shoulder Roll stretch, you're using the muscles in each shoulder to move your shoulder through its full range of motion and stretch its muscles.

Benefits
* Relieves tension through the upper traps, rhomboids, and deltoids.
* Improves shoulder mobility and function, guarding against common shoulder restrictions.
* Trains the rotator cuff muscles and connective tissues.
* Helps ease the kyphosis (rounded upper spine) that can occur with frequent computer, tablet, and phone use, as well as with aging.
* Improves form during upper-body exercises such as rows and presses.

Steps:

1. Squeeze your upper traps to raise your shoulders toward your ears.
2. Keeping your shoulders raised, squeeze your shoulder blades to shift your shoulders behind your body.
3. Squeeze your shoulder blades down to lower your shoulders to your sides.
4. Squeeze your chest to shift your shoulders in front of your body.
5. Keeping your shoulders in front of your body, squeeze your upper traps to raise your shoulders toward your ears.
6. Complete the number of reps that work for you, then switch directions.

To Deepen This Stretch...

* Let your upper back arch, then curl forward with each roll.

Shoulder Rotation

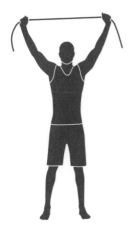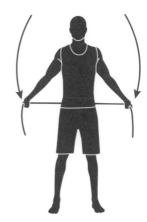

Shoulder Rotation is one of the best dynamic shoulder stretches you can do before working out because it takes your shoulder joints through their full 360-degree range of motion. This stretch gets blood to the joints, warms up your postural muscles, and helps you do practically any exercise or movement with better form. The key here, especially if you choose to deepen the stretch with a resistance band or dowel, is to avoid leaning your shoulders back or arching your lower back. While leaning your shoulders back or arching your lower back can make it easier to achieve hard-to-reach shoulder positions, this doesn't benefit your shoulders and can actually stress your lower back.

Benefits

* Relieves tension through and warms up the upper traps and deltoids.
* Improves shoulder mobility and function, guarding against common shoulder restrictions.

* Trains the rotator cuff muscles and connective tissues.
* Improves form during both upper-body and lower-body exercises that involve holding a weight.

Steps:
1. Hold one end of a resistance band, rope, or dowel in each hand, with your hands roughly double shoulder-width apart and your arms extended in front of your thighs.
2. Raise your arms overhead and then behind you to the back of your hips.
3. Pause, then raise your arms overhead and then down diagonally in front of your thighs.

To Deepen This Stretch...
* Hold the band or dowel with your hands closer to each other.

Butterfly

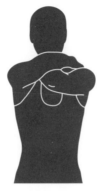

Here's a feel-good shoulder stretch you most likely haven't tried. This stretch really isolates the rear deltoids to give these often-missed muscles the attention they need. This stretch is quick and simple, and it takes up hardly any space, meaning it's easy to do whenever the moment strikes, like when you're at your desk or commuting to work. If during this stretch you feel any discomfort or hear creaking in the front of your shoulders, try dropping your elbows to your chest.

Benefits
* Relieves tension through the rear (posterior) deltoid, teres minor, and supraspinatus in the back of the shoulder.
* Helps ease the kyphosis (rounded upper spine) that can occur with frequent computer, tablet, and phone use, as well as with aging.
* Improves shoulder mobility and function, guarding against common shoulder restrictions.

Steps:
1. Place your palms on opposite shoulders, with your elbows raised straight in front of you.

2. Squeeze through the front of your shoulders and chest to stack your elbows on top of each other.
3. Hold.

To Deepen This Stretch...
* Once your elbows are stacked, round your shoulders and pull your upper arms forward away from your body.

Band Pull-Apart

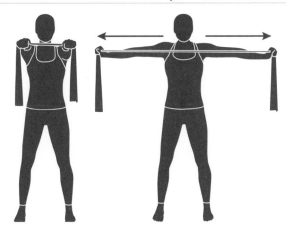

This dynamic stretch benefits the muscles surrounding your shoulder blades, especially if you're gearing up for an upper-body workout or have any neck pain. That's because it's one of the most effective ways to correct rounded shoulders and posture—simultaneously stretching and strengthening the muscles that keep your posture upright. Try this stretch whenever you need to release tension or before an upper-body workout or any activity that requires stable shoulders. For the greatest benefits, concentrate on making all movement come from your shoulders. Your torso, elbows, and wrists should stay completely stationary.

Benefits

* Relieves tension through and warms up the upper traps, rhomboids, rotator cuff muscles, and rear deltoids.
* Trains the rotator cuff muscles and connective tissues.

* Helps ease the kyphosis (rounded upper spine) that can occur with frequent computer, tablet, and phone use, as well as with aging.
* Improves form during upper-body exercises such as rows and presses.

Steps:

1. Hold a resistance band straight out in front of your shoulders with both hands.
2. Squeeze your shoulder blades together to move your arms straight out to your sides in a T shape.
3. Pause, then slowly bring your arms back in front of you with control.

To Deepen This Stretch...

* Hold the band with your hands closer to each other.

Overhead Triceps

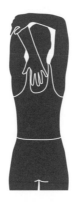

Your triceps contain three muscle segments, called "heads." The biggest and longest of the three is aptly called the long head, or triceps longus. It starts at your shoulder blade and runs all the way to your ulna, a bone in your forearm. This stretch works the long head at both ends, putting the muscle in a fully stretched position that's not possible with non-overhead triceps stretches.

Benefits
* Relieves tension through the triceps as well as the teres minor and major in the back of the shoulder.
* Addresses the hard-to-reach triceps longus, which connects to the shoulder joint.
* Maintains and improves healthy range of motion in the shoulder and elbow.
* Improves form during upper-body exercises such as shoulder presses.

Steps:

1. Raise one arm overhead and bend that elbow, dropping the forearm between your shoulder blades.
2. With your other hand, grab your upper arm just above your bent elbow.
3. Gently pull your elbow toward your ear and your arm down your back.

To Deepen This Stretch...

* Lean your torso away from your raised arm.

Seated Biceps

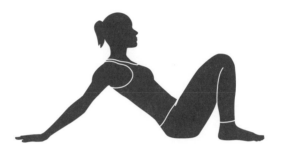

The biceps aren't the easiest muscles to target during your stretching routine. Fortunately, this stretch helps you target them in a creative way. By placing your arms behind you and straightening your elbows, you'll work the biceps from their two attachment points—your shoulders and elbows. To get the greatest benefit from this stretch, work to bring your arms as far and straight behind you as possible without being uncomfortable.

Benefits
* Relieves tension through the biceps brachii, brachialis, and brachioradialis muscles as well as the anterior deltoid and pectoralis major.
* Helps ease the rounded shoulders that can occur with frequent computer, tablet, and phone use, as well as with aging.
* Maintains and improves healthy range of motion in the shoulder and elbow.
* Can improve strength for pulling exercises such as rows and pull-ups (when done dynamically and very gently).

Steps:

1. Sit on the floor with your feet flat and knees bent.
2. Place your palms on the floor behind you, shoulder-width apart, with your fingers pointing away from you.
3. Keeping your hands in place, slowly slide your hips forward and away from your hands. Lock your elbows so the creases of your elbows point to your hips rather than the sides.

To Deepen This Stretch...

* Slide your hips farther from your hands.

Doorway Pec

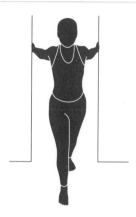

When people have tight or rounded shoulders, the first thing they usually do is stretch their upper back. And while that certainly can help, leaving the chest unstretched is a big mistake. That's because the chest muscles—the pectoralis major and minor—connect to your upper arm bone and your ribs, right by your collarbone, respectively. Because your day's activities are all done in front of your body, your chest muscles can pull your shoulder muscles forward, causing an unhealthy tugging on your upper-back muscles.

Benefits
* Relieves tension through the pectoralis major and minor, anterior deltoids, biceps brachii, brachialis, and brachioradialis muscles.
* Helps ease tightness in the front of the chest and shoulders that can contribute to rounded shoulders.
* Reduces how hard the upper-back muscles are stretched during everyday activities by relaxing contracted muscles in front of the shoulders.

* Improves form during both upper-body and lower-body exercises that involve holding a weight (when done dynamically).

Steps:
1. Stand in the center of a doorway and place your palms on both sides of the door frame.
2. Step forward a couple of feet with one foot.
3. Lean forward through your torso.

To Deepen This Stretch...
* Stretch each arm separately, standing next to a wall instead of in a doorway. Place one hand on the wall behind you, then slowly step closer to the wall until you feel a gentle stretch in your chest and front of your shoulder. Hold, then switch sides. Progress to extend your arm straight behind you.

Wrist Flexion and Extension

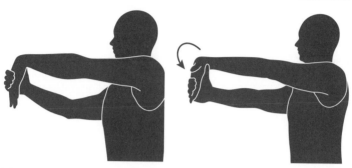

Throughout the day, your wrists usually stay in a neutral position, with your hands more or less in line with your forearms. While this is a healthy placement for your wrist—and ideal for any ergonomic desk setup—it's beneficial to move your wrist joints through their full available range of motion. That includes flexing your wrists to draw your palms toward your forearms as well as extending them to draw the back of your hands to your forearms. The finger flexors in the front of your forearm tend to be the tightest, while the finger extensors are often the weaker of the two groups.

Benefits

* Relieves tension through the finger flexors in the front of the forearm and the finger extensors in the back of the forearm.
* Expands wrist mobility and dexterity during both everyday and athletic feats of strength.
* Warms up the wrist joints and forearm muscles before grip-heavy exercises like dead lifts and rock climbing (when done dynamically).
* Makes exercises that require full wrist extension more comfortable, such as push-ups and high planks (when done statically).

Steps:
1. Extend one arm straight in front of your shoulder with your palm facing down. Keep your elbow straight.
2. Place your other hand on the back of your extended hand. Gently press down to bend your wrist so your fingers point down.
3. Hold, then release and rotate your extended arm so that your palm faces up.
4. Place your other hand at the base of your extended hand's fingers. Gently press down to extend your wrist so your fingers point down.
5. Hold, then release. Complete the number of reps that work for you, then switch arms.

To Deepen This Stretch...
* Instead of placing your helping hand on the back of your extended hand and then the base of your fingers, put that hand on the back of your knuckles and then on the ends of your fingers.

Figure 8

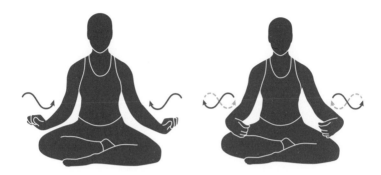

Your wrists move in more directions than back-and-forth; they also move from side to side or around in circles. This dynamic stretch moves your wrists through their full range of motion, improving joint mobility and increasing blood flow to the area. Try the Figure 8 stretch before your workouts (like lifting, tennis, climbing, etc.) and throughout the day. This stretch is especially effective if your wrists are often restricted or give you any pain.

Benefits

* Relieves tension through the finger flexors, finger extensors, and small stabilizing muscles of the forearms and wrists.
* Expands wrist mobility and dexterity during both everyday and athletic feats of strength.
* Warms up the wrist joints and forearm muscles before grip-heavy exercises like dead lifts and rock climbing.
* Makes it more comfortable to do exercises that require full wrist extension, such as push-ups and high planks (when done statically).

Steps:

1. Make relaxed fists with both hands, with your palms facing down.
2. Roll your wrists in figure 8 or "infinity" shapes. Your palms should alternate between facing up and down as you move through the shape.
3. With each roll, try to make the 8 shape bigger.

To Deepen This Stretch...

* Clasp both hands together, interlacing your fingers and pressing your palms into each other. Complete your rolls from this position, gently pressing each hand into the other.

Open-Hand Wrist Rotation

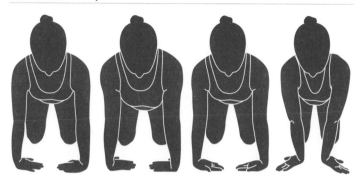

An advanced combination of the Wrist Flexion and Extension and the Figure 8 stretches, this stretch gives the area from your forearms to your elbows an intense stretch. Try it once you feel comfortable with the previous wrist stretches and are ready to challenge yourself. Throughout this stretch, listen to your body and only rotate your wrists as far as feels comfortable.

Benefits

* Relieves tension through the finger flexors in the front of the forearm and the finger extensors in the back of the forearm.
* Expands wrist mobility and dexterity during both everyday and athletic feats of strength.
* Warms up the wrist joint and forearm muscles before grip-heavy exercises like dead lifts and rock climbing (when done dynamically).
* Makes it more comfortable to do exercises that require full wrist extension, such as push-ups and high planks (when done statically).

Steps:

1. From a kneeling position, place your palms flat on the floor with your fingers pointed toward each other and your elbows straight.
2. Keeping your palms on the floor, rotate your wrists a full 360 degrees until your fingers again point toward each other and your elbows face each other. (Note: If you can't do the full rotation, just do as much you can.)
3. Move back-and-forth between the two positions.
4. Complete the number of reps that work for you, then repeat with the backs of your hands on the floor.

To Deepen This Stretch...

*   Gradually shift your body weight into your arms.

Wrist Flexion with Finger Touch

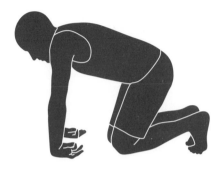

This stretch trains both wrist flexibility and mobility as well as finger dexterity. This stretch also improves your body's proprioception. Often called the "sixth sense," proprioception is the neurological ability to know where your body parts are and how they're moving, without having to look at them. Improving this ability means better finger control and coordination. Want to play the piano, become a better typist, or make it to the top of the rock-climbing wall? Then practice this stretch.

Benefits
* Relieves tension through the finger extensors in the back of the forearm.
* Improves finger dexterity and coordination.
* Warms up the wrist joint and forearm muscles before grip-heavy exercises like dead lifts and rock climbing.
* Makes it more comfortable to do exercises that require full wrist extension, such as push-ups and high planks (when done statically).

Steps:

1. From a kneeling position, place the backs of your hands on the floor with your fingers pointed toward your body and your elbows straight.
2. Keeping your hands on the floor, touch your thumb to your index finger.
3. Repeat, touching your thumb to each of your other three fingers.

To Deepen This Stretch...

* Sit back into your hips so your hands are farther in front of your body.

Joint-by-Joint Finger Flexion and Extension

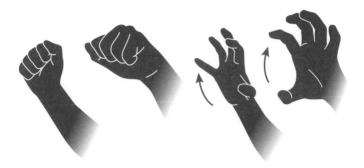

Your fingers have a vast array of tendons and ligaments (and nerves!) that can benefit from stretching. Since these tissues connect to your arm bones and joints, moving your fingers through their full range of motion positively affects your entire arms.

Benefits
* Relieves tension through the tissues of the hands and fingers.
* Trains neuromuscular control and coordination of the fingers.
* Expands finger mobility and dexterity during both everyday and athletic feats of strength.
* Moves blood into the fingers to warm up their joints.

Steps:
1. Make tight fists with both hands.
2. Slowly, joint by joint, uncurl your fingers until they are fully extended behind your palms.
3. Slowly, starting at the tips of your fingers, reverse the motion to curl your fingers back into a tight fist.

To Deepen This Stretch...
* As you extend your fingers, also spread them out and away from each other.

Child's Pose

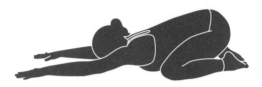

Everybody's favorite yoga pose, Child's Pose is a relaxing way to ease tension in the muscles spanning from your shoulder blades into your lower back. And even if you're focusing on your back, you can rest comfortably knowing this pose opens up your hips and inner thighs. During this stretch, your goal is to relax your muscles as much as possible. Resist the urge to contract anything. Let gravity pull your body down into the position that's right for you. This will help you capitalize on the stretch's mental and emotional health benefits.

Benefits
* Relieves tension through the rotator cuffs, upper and lower traps, lats, and lower back.
* Maintains and improves healthy range of motion in the spine, shoulders, and hips.
* Calms the mind and relieves stress.
* Relaxes the posterior chain (low back, gluteals, hamstrings, and calves) after back-focused workouts and sports.

Steps:

1. Get on your hands and knees with your legs just farther than shoulder-width apart.
2. Keeping your hands in place, sit your hips back toward the floor between your feet.
3. Bend your torso forward and rest your forehead onto the floor.

To Deepen This Stretch...

* As you hold the stretch, walk your hands to one side, then the other.

Thread-the-Needle

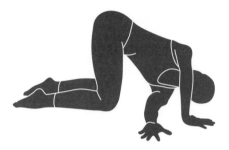

This yoga-inspired stretch works to untwist the knots most people have in their upper backs and shoulders. Remember, the goal isn't to prove your flexibility but simply to stretch your muscles. Once you have moved into position, focus on relaxing all of your body's muscles to help you fully sink into the stretch and reduce any discomfort that can occur with resistance. Try this stretch dynamically before workouts or statically at the end of the day to improve your sleep.

Benefits

* Relieves tension through the rotator cuffs, rhomboids, upper and lower traps, lats, and lower back.
* Maintains and improves healthy range of motion in the spine and shoulders.
* Calms the mind and relieves stress.
* Relaxes the posterior chain (low back, gluteals, hamstrings, and calves) after back-focused workouts and sports.

Steps:

1. Get on your hands and knees with your knees under your hips and hands under your shoulders.
2. Turn one hand to place the back of it on the floor with your fingers pointed toward your other hand.

3. Slide your hand across the floor underneath and then past your planted arm's side.
4. Rotate your torso and lower your upper back and head against the floor.
5. Hold, then switch sides.

To Deepen This Stretch...
  * Extend your arm and walk your planted hand above your head on the floor.
  * As you breathe, imagine trying to inflate the stretched muscles.

Standing Lat Dive

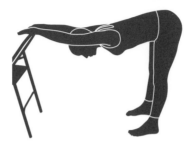

Somewhat like a standing Child's Pose, this stretch targets many of the same muscles, including your lats and traps. Unlike Child's Pose, however, this stretch is not something to simply relax into. By taking a standing position, you're able to extend your thoracic spine more than is possible during Child's Pose, and you can actively work to press your torso toward the floor. In other words, you get a deeper stretch in the middle of your back.

Benefits
* Relieves tension through the rotator cuffs, upper and lower traps, lats, and lower back.
* Maintains and improves healthy range of motion in the spine, shoulders, and hips.
* Improves form during upper-body exercises such as rows and presses (when done dynamically).
* Relaxes the posterior chain (low back, gluteals, hamstrings, and calves) after back-focused workouts and sports (when done statically).

Steps:

1. Place your hands on the back of a chair, standing far enough away that you can extend your arms straight in front of you.
2. Push your hips back behind you and slightly bend your knees, lowering your torso forward until it's parallel with the floor.

To Deepen This Stretch...

* Actively press your chest toward the floor to lower your torso past your hands.

Wall Slide

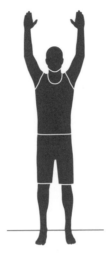

It looks easy, but this dynamic stretch requires (and, fortunately, builds) greater mobility through your back and shoulders. This stretch focuses on upward shoulder rotation: teaching your rotator cuff muscles how to control your shoulder blades as they flare to the sides to help raise your arms straight overhead. Upward shoulder rotation is a movement pattern that nearly every person struggles with in some form, and that contributes to both shoulder restrictions and, most noticeably, lower-back pain. After all, if your upper back lacks the mobility it needs, your body is going to make up for it—by excessively arching and stressing your lumbar spine.

Benefits

* Relieves tension through the upper and lower traps, lats, rhomboids, and deltoids.
* Improves spinal and shoulder mobility and alignment.
* Trains the rotator cuff muscles and connective tissues.

* Helps ease the kyphosis (rounded upper spine) that can occur with frequent computer, tablet, and phone use, as well as with aging.
* Improves form during upper-body exercises, especially those that involve overhead work.

Steps:

1. Stand with your back, hips, and head against a wall.
2. Step your feet about a foot away from the wall to lean some of your weight into the wall.
3. Bend your elbows and press the back of your arms against the wall to mimic a goalpost.
4. Keeping your back, hips, and head against the wall—and minimizing any arch in your lower back—slowly straighten your arms to slide them up the wall overhead.

To Deepen This Stretch...

* Actively press your arms into the wall.

T-Spine Extension

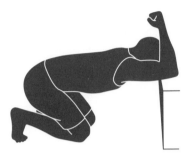

This stretch is all about improving flexibility and mobility in and around the T, or thoracic, spine. Daily life requires the T-spine to spend a lot of time in a forward-flexed position. By targeting the opposing action—extension—performing this gentle movement can help open up your back muscles, improve spinal alignment, and help your body work and move more efficiently during virtually anything you do. This stretch also helps to relax the muscles in the middle of your back and shoulders.

Benefits
* Relieves tension through the rotator cuffs, upper and lower traps, lats, and lower back.
* Maintains and improves healthy range of motion in the spine, shoulders, and hips.
* Helps ease the kyphosis (rounded upper spine) that can occur with frequent computer, tablet, and phone use, as well as with aging.
* Improves form during upper-body exercises, especially those that involve overhead work.

Steps:

1. Kneel next to a bench and hold a dowel or resistance band with your hands shoulder-width apart and palms facing up.
2. Bend your elbows and place them on top of the bench with your shoulders, elbows, and wrists in line with each other.
3. Sit your hips back toward your heels and let your torso fall toward the floor.

To Deepen This Stretch...

* Hold the stretch for more time.
* On each exhale, actively press your torso lower toward the floor.

T-Spine Rotation

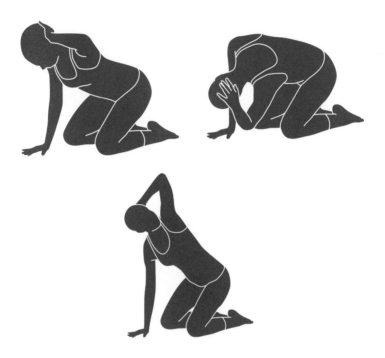

This dynamic stretch is a wonderful pre-workout exercise that simul-taneously loosens and activates the muscles that connect to your T-spine. This stretch also improves the flow of blood and nutrients to your spine, which improves your ability to fully rotate through your T-spine. When stretching your T-spine, you'll find it easier to do every-day motions like reaching behind you to your car's back seat, as well as gym exercises like woodchops.

Benefits

 * Relieves tension through the rotator cuffs, upper and lower traps, lats, and lower back.
 * Maintains and improves healthy range of motion in the spine, shoulders, and hips.
 * Promotes the flow of blood, oxygen, and nutrients to the spine and neighboring, otherwise blood-poor, tissues.
 * Improves form during upper-body exercises, especially those that involve overhead work.

Steps:

1. Get on your hands and knees with your spine in a neutral position.
2. Place one hand on the back of your head, pointing your elbow straight out to your side.
3. Keeping your elbow in line with your torso, rotate your torso to drop your elbow to point down straight to the floor.
4. Reverse the motion to raise your elbow to point straight up to the ceiling.

To Deepen This Stretch...

 * At the bottom of the pose, try to point your elbow to your planted hand. At the top, try to point your elbow behind you.
 * Hold each position a little longer each time.

Supine Spinal Twist

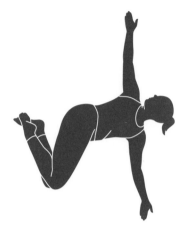

This stretch is similar to the T-Spine Rotation, but rather than requiring you to actively work and squeeze your muscles, it takes full advantage of gravity's downward pull, so all you have to do is relax into the twist. This might not boost blood flow through your back, or really help you warm up prior to exercise, but it's a helpful static stretch for relaxation, such as before bedtime. Plus, this stretch brings your hips farther into the equation, helping you improve mobility through your sacrum, the bottom part of your spine that connects to your pelvis.

Benefits
* Relieves tension through the rotator cuffs, upper and lower traps, lats, and lower back.
* Maintains and improves healthy range of motion in the spine, shoulders, and hips.
* Relaxes the mind and body.
* Improves form during upper-body exercises, especially those that involve overhead work.

Steps:
1. Lie on your back with your knees bent and feet flat on the floor. Relax your arms straight out to your sides with your palms facing up.
2. Drop your knees to one side until they reach the floor.
3. Turn your head and upper back to face the opposite side of your knees. Try to keep both shoulder blades flat against the floor.
4. Hold, then switch sides.

To Deepen This Stretch...
* Place one hand on your knees to actively press them down against the floor.
* Rotate your head and upper back from side to side, placing your hands together and then spreading them out wide. Imagine you're opening and closing a book.

I-Y-T-A

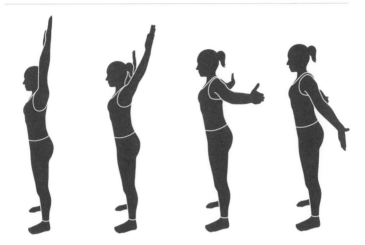

You have a seemingly infinite number of little muscles wrapping around and connecting your shoulder blades to your spine and each other. This dynamic stretch is one of the best ways to both contract and elongate these muscles. This stretch is especially beneficial before any workouts or sports that involve pulling or pushing through your upper body. In each position, you should feel an intense pressure between your shoulder blades, almost like a massage therapist is working on your muscles. If you feel too much pressure or discomfort, stop, shake your arms out, and then try again, while focusing on keeping your back straight and moving your arms solely by pinching through your shoulder blades.

Benefits

* Relieves tension through and warms up the upper and lower traps, lats, rhomboids, and rotator cuff muscles.
* Helps ease the kyphosis (rounded upper spine) that can occur with frequent computer, tablet, and phone use, as well as with aging.

* Promotes the flow of blood, oxygen, and nutrients to the spine and neighboring, otherwise blood-poor, tissues.
* Improves form and strength during upper-body exercises such as rows and presses, as well as any move that involves holding a weight.
* Reduces the risk of back aches and pains during exercise.

Steps:

1. Extend your arms above your head with your palms facing forward.
2. Moving only from your shoulders and, without arching through your lower back, squeeze your shoulder blades together to pull your arms back behind your shoulders in an I shape. Release.
3. Repeat with your arms positioned in a Y (arms diagonally overhead), a T (arms straight out to your sides), and an A (arms diagonally to your sides).

To Deepen This Stretch...

* Hold each position statically. Stand in the middle of a doorway, and grasp the frame with both hands to help you hold each position.

Rounded-Back Knee Pull

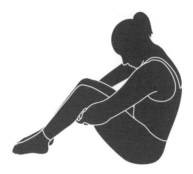

This assisted motion—meaning it uses props (in this case, your knees) to help you gain leverage and stretch your muscles to their max—is ideal for when you really want to work your middle- and upper-back muscles. By holding under your knees during this stretch, you're able to flex your thoracic spine more than you can by simply bending forward. Try this stretch throughout the day at your desk, after workouts as a relaxing cooldown, or before bed to let go of the day's stress and tension.

Benefits

* Relieves tension through the upper and lower traps, lats, rhomboids, and rotator cuff muscles.
* Maintains and improves healthy range of motion in the thoracic spine and shoulders.
* Undoes the upper-back tension that comes with repetitive forward-facing activities like driving, typing, running, and cycling.
* Relaxes the posterior chain (low back, gluteals, hamstrings, and calves) after back-focused workouts and sports.

Steps:

1. Sit on the floor with your knees bent and feet flat on the floor in front of you, spread shoulder-width apart.
2. Wrap your arms around the outsides of your thighs and grab your wrists under your knees.
3. Lean your torso back and arch your spine. Don't let your legs, your anchor point, move.

To Deepen This Stretch...

* Try it with a partner, each of you holding the same rope or long, looped resistance band with your hands shoulder-width apart. As you lean back, have your partner gently pull on the rope to "fight" your pull.

Pelvic Tilt

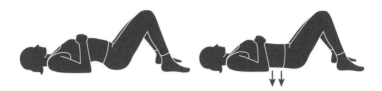

The perfect combination of a lower-back stretch and core-strengthening exercise, the Pelvic Tilt helps correct both mild and severe anterior pelvic tilt. In fact, the stretch is as simple as tilting your pelvis posteriorly, relaxing, and then doing it again. This stretch teaches you how to properly tilt your pelvis posteriorly. During each flow (a smooth movement between stretches), you gently relieve compression on the lumbar vertebrae and their discs, relax your lower-back muscles, and learn how to use your core to properly align your pelvis with the rest of your spine.

Benefits
* Relieves tension through the erector spinae, lower-back muscles, and connective tissues surrounding the lumbar spine.
* Reduces compression on the lumbar vertebrae and their discs.
* Maintains and improves healthy range of motion in the lumbar spine and pelvis.
* Eases lower-back pain due to lordosis (inward curving of lower back) and spinal and pelvic alignment issues.

Steps:
1. Lie faceup with your feet flat on the floor, hip-width apart. There should be space between your lower back and the floor.
2. Squeeze your abs to tighten your core and tuck your tailbone to press your lower back against the floor.
3. Hold, then slowly reverse the motion.

To Deepen This Stretch...
* Hold for more time, or as long as you can without letting your lower back lose contact with the floor.
* Press through your heels to raise your hips from the floor as high as possible.

Standing Reach

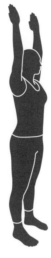

This simple static stretch focuses on lengthening the spine, reducing pressure between the vertebrae, and releasing downward and forward tension through the core muscles and tissues. An effective but very gentle stretch, it's a great place to start any core-stretching routine or exercise warm-up. This stretch eases your body into the movements to come in your workout while reinforcing strong, healthy posture. If you choose to enhance the stretch with a slight backward bend, focus on doing so while still maintaining a tall, elongated spine. Use your muscles to actively lift your weight upward, rather than letting it settle onto your lower back.

Benefits

* Relieves tension through the transverse abdominis, rectus abdominis, serratus anterior, and erector spinae.
* Reduces any excess forward pull of the rectus abdominis on the spine.
* Helps relax the shoulders down and away from the ears for better posture.
* Improves form during both standing and seated exercises.
* Readies the body for more intense core stretches.

Steps:

1. Stand with your feet hip-width apart and your arms at your sides. Brace your core.
2. Without arching your lower back or hunching up your shoulders toward your ears, raise your arms straight up overhead.
3. Reach as high as possible, leading with your fingertips. Simultaneously soften your knees, press through your feet, and brace your legs to stabilize and engage your lower body.

To Deepen This Stretch...

* Squeeze your glutes and slowly point your arms and torso just behind your body.

Cat-Cow

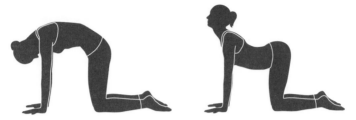

Cat-Cow is one of the most basic and popular yoga poses, but you don't need to be a yogi to reap its benefits. By moving between two opposite spinal postures, you alternate between stretching the front and then the back muscles of your core, with one muscle group lengthening, and the other contracting, which boosts blood flow through your torso. Plus, as the back-and-forth motion gently massages your gut, this stretch helps promote healthy digestion and relieves stress.

Benefits

* Relieves tension through the transverse abdominis, rectus abdominis, serratus anterior, latissimus dorsi, pectorals, and erector spinae. This stretch also engages and stretches the hip flexors and hip extensors (in the front and back of the hips).
* Reduces any excess forward pull of the rectus abdominis on the spine.
* Eases lower-back pain.
* Helps relax the shoulders down and away from the ears for better posture.
* Calms the mind and body.

Steps:

1. Get on your hands and knees with your knees under your hips and your wrists under your shoulders.
2. Slowly exhale, tucking your tailbone toward the floor and dropping your chin to your chest. Let your back round toward the ceiling. This is the Cat position.
3. Slowly inhale, pointing your tailbone toward the ceiling while raising your chin. Let your back round toward the floor. This is the Cow position.

To Deepen This Stretch...

* Hold each position for a few seconds.

Sphinx

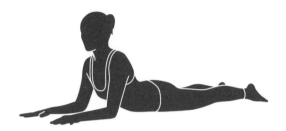

Another yoga-inspired stretch, Sphinx is similar to the Cow portion of Cat-Cow because it lifts and bends the muscles at the front of the core to combat forward-leaning postures and help you avoid the upper-back rounding known as kyphosis. This "lifting" component of the stretch is vital, especially if you have a history of lower-back aches and pains. Sphinx will also provide relief to the small of your back if you lead the stretch by opening your chest and abs. However, if you move passively through the stretch, resting your body weight in your arms, you can unwittingly "dump" your torso's weight into the small of your back. This stretch looks simple, but don't let that be a reason to take your focus off of form.

Benefits
* Relieves tension through the transverse abdominis, rectus abdominis, pectorals, and deltoids.
* Reduces any excess forward pull of the rectus abdominis and pectorals on the spine.
* Eases lower-back pain.
* Helps relax the shoulders down and away from the ears for better posture.
* Energizes the mind and body.

Steps:

1. Lie facedown on the floor with your legs straight behind you. Place your elbows under your shoulders with your forearms flat on the floor.
2. Press the tops of your feet into the floor.
3. Slowly inhale, pressing your forearms, pelvis, and tops of your feet against the floor to raise your head and chest toward the ceiling. Gently squeeze your shoulder blades down and together.
4. Hold. To release, exhale and lower your chest back to the floor.

To Deepen This Stretch...

* Straighten your elbows and press through your hands to raise your chest higher toward the ceiling.

Seated Side Bend

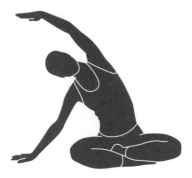

Most people have tried some version of this side stretch. Most people, however, tend to bend forward while bending to the side. In this stretch, you'll focus on only moving to the side. Your torso, chest, and head will point straight forward at all times—as if your core, chest, and arms are sandwiched between two panes of glass. By not bending your torso forward, you'll focus on stretching the muscles of your sides, rather than your back.

Benefits

* Relieves tension through the serratus anterior and obliques.
* Eases lower-back pain.
* Improves form during upper-body exercises and lower-body exercises that require holding a weight or twisting through the torso.
* Both calms and energizes the mind and body.

Steps:

1. Sit tall on the floor or in a chair with your shoulders down and hands at your sides.
2. Raise one arm overhead and lean your torso to the opposite side of your raised arm, keeping your other hand on the floor for support.
3. Hold, using each inhale to deepen the stretch. Switch sides.

To Deepen This Stretch...

* Stand up and let the stretch extend into your hip.

Serratus Roll

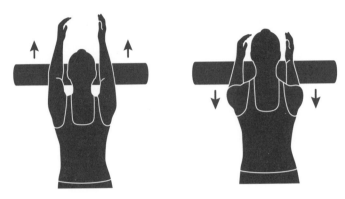

It's time to get to know your serratus anterior. There are other stretches in this section that work this muscle, but this stretch really focuses on it. The SA, sometimes called "the boxer's muscle," is what helps you punch, or outstretch, your arms in front of you. Running down your sides, this muscle attaches your ribs to your shoulder blades. The Serratus Roll simultaneously stretches and strengthens the SA—both of which are necessary to keep the upper half of your core mobile and in good alignment.

Benefits

* Relieves tension through and warms up the serratus anterior.
* Strengthens the transverse abdominis.
* Stretches the sides of the core.
* Improves form during upper-body exercises such as rows and presses.

Steps:

1. Stand a foot or so in front of a wall and place the sides of your forearms against a foam roller at chest height with your thumbs facing you. Your elbows and wrists should be in line with your shoulders.
2. Squeeze your shoulders forward toward the wall to create a slight hunch in your upper back.
3. Slowly extend your shoulders and elbows to roll the foam roller up the wall as high as possible while keeping your shoulders rounded forward.
4. Pause, then slowly roll back down.

To Deepen This Stretch...

* Hold the top position for more time.
* Loop a mini resistance band around your forearms. Don't let the band pull your arms together throughout the stretch.

Overhead Curl

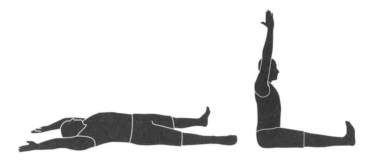

This dynamic, advanced stretch strengthens the core, but don't confuse it with a crunch or quiver-inducing abdominal exercise. While doing this stretch, your focus should be on moving slowly and deliberately from vertebrae to vertebrae. This move requires a base level of core strength. If you have trouble with it, try the range of motion with a solid form. With time and practice, that range of motion will grow.

Benefits
* Relieves tension through and warms up the transverse abdominis, rectus abdominis, serratus anterior, latissimus dorsi, and erector spinae.
* Lengthens the spine to reduce pressure between the vertebrae and promote good spinal alignment. (You may hear a crack or two.)
* Massages the back muscles.
* Calms the mind and body.

Steps:

1. Lie faceup on the floor with your arms and legs fully extended. Reach through your arms and legs to pull yourself long (while keeping your shoulders down and away from your ears). Brace your core by tucking in your tailbone to press your lower back into the floor.

2. Keeping this stretch, slowly exhale and curl your spine up and forward until you're sitting straight up and your arms are vertical, stretched high toward the ceiling. Round through your shoulders and then down to your lower back.

3. Slowly inhale and lower down to the floor, curling your spine with your arms overhead. Round through your lower back and then up to your shoulders.

To Deepen This Stretch…

* Lower your back as slowly as possible.

Seated Twist

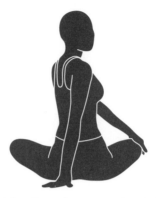

One very important function of your core is rotational movement—twisting from side to side. Your internal and external obliques control this type of movement. If you don't spend time practicing this twist, your movement can become limited. By taking your spine through its full rotational range of motion, you relax the obliques while stretching any stiffness near the spine that might prevent you from twisting. To do this stretch, keep your eyes on the goal: rotating through your entire torso, not just your shoulders. Resist the urge to use your arms to try to press yourself into a deeper twist. Actively squeeze your core and back muscles to find your end range of motion. Then use your arms to firm up and stabilize the position.

Benefits
* Relieves tension through the latissimus dorsi, serratus anterior, obliques, and lower back.
* Opens the upper back and shoulders while strengthening the hips and legs.
* Maintains and improves healthy rotational movement of the spine.
* Calms the mind and relieves stress.

Steps:

1. Sit on the floor with your legs crossed. Extend the top of your head tall toward the ceiling.
2. Place one hand on the opposite knee and the other on the floor behind you.
3. Focusing on staying as tall as possible, rotate your torso toward your back hand.
4. Hold, then switch sides.

To Deepen This Stretch...

* Keeping one leg crossed in front of your body, place your other foot flat on the floor with that leg's knee pointed toward the ceiling. Extend one arm and place it against the outside of the opposite bent knee. Place your other hand on the floor behind you and rotate as before.

Chair Twist

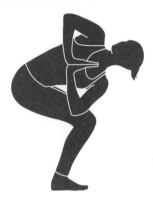

Another rotational stretch, this provides a great opportunity to challenge yourself to include your hips and shoulders. Expect to feel a stretch through your back, abs, and shoulders as well as a contraction through your glutes and quads. The longer you hold the stretch, the more you turn it into a feat of lower-body strength. Tailor your pacing to fit your goals.

Benefits

* Relieves tension through the latissimus dorsi, serratus anterior, obliques, and lower back.
* Engages the shoulder and hip muscles.
* Maintains and improves healthy rotational movement of the spine.
* Both calms and energizes the mind and body.

Steps:

1. Stand tall with your feet together. Squeeze your abs to brace your core.
2. Push your hips back behind you and bend your knees as if you are sitting in an invisible chair.

3. Place your palms together with your elbows out to your sides.
4. Keeping your hips and knees stacked, slowly exhale, and rotate your torso down and to one side. Your elbows should be in a vertical line. Place your bottom elbow against the outside of your knees.
5. Hold, using each inhale to deepen the stretch. To release, inhale and rotate to face forward. Straighten, then switch sides.

To Deepen This Stretch...

* Hold for more time.
* Turn your head to face the ceiling.
* Once in the stretch, extend your bottom arm toward the floor and your top arm toward the ceiling.

Contralateral Limb Raise

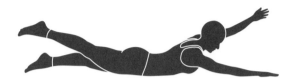

This dynamic stretch works the anterior core, strengthens the hips and back, improves coordination, and teaches you how to create total-body tension (read: squeezing every muscle from head to toe). Total-body tension takes advantage of your body's ability to work as a single unit with no "weak link" to be found. This improves how effectively and efficiently you perform any given task while keeping your spine and joints in healthy alignment with each other. For the greatest benefit, focus on actively squeezing your posterior core muscles to raise your limbs, rather than lifting them up and then relying on your lower-back arch to hold them there. With each repetition, raise only as high as you can without any discomfort to your lower back.

Benefits
* Relieves tension through the transverse abdominis, rectus abdominis, pectorals, and deltoids.
* Reduces excess forward pull of the rectus abdominis and pectorals on the spine.
* Strengthens the glutes as well as the lower and upper back.
* Eases lower-back pain.
* Improves form during both standing and seated exercises.

Steps:

1. Lie facedown on the floor with your arms and legs fully extended. Reach through both your arms and legs to pull yourself long. Squeeze your abs to brace your core.
2. Squeeze your glutes and upper back to raise one arm and the opposite leg about a foot off of the floor.
3. Pause, then slowly lower your arm and leg to the floor. Alternate sides with each repetition.

To Deepen This Stretch...

* Hold each arm and leg raise for more time.
* Raise both arms, and only your arms, with each repetition.
* Raise both legs, and only your legs, with each repetition.
* Raise both arms and both legs with each repetition.

Glute Bridge

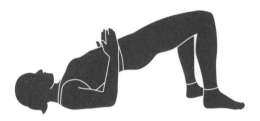

A common hip-strengthening move, this stretch is a great way to relieve tension through the hip flexors and lower fibers of the anterior core. When these muscles are tight, they pull your torso down toward the front of your pelvis and the front of your pelvis up toward your torso, encouraging lordosis, which is excessive inward curvature of the spine. Whether you move quickly between repetitions or hold the stretch for fifteen, thirty, or even sixty seconds, make it a priority to squeeze your glutes and hips as tight as possible during this stretch. This will increase the stretch through both your hip flexors and the front of your core.

Benefits
* Relieves tension through the hip flexors as well as the lower fibers of the transverse abdominis and rectus abdominis.
* Reduces excess forward pull of the rectus abdominis on the spine.
* Eases lower-back pain.
* Strengthens the gluteus maximus.
* Improves form during lower-body exercises by warming up the glutes and hips.

Steps:

1. Lie faceup with your back, hips, and feet flat on the floor, hip-width apart.

2. Anchor your upper arms into the floor beside you. Squeeze your core and tuck your tailbone to press your lower back into the floor.

3. Press your heels into the floor and squeeze your glutes to raise your hips until your torso forms a straight line from your knees to shoulders.

4. Hold.

To Deepen This Stretch...

* Relax your core and raise your abdomen toward the ceiling, letting your back arch.

90-90

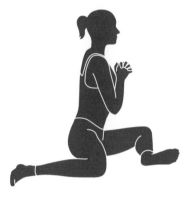

The 90-90 stretch is a great way to improve your hip flexibility and mobility at the same time. While most hip stretches focus only on stretching either internal or external hip rotation, this stretch does both, giving you a complete hip stretch in one position. This stretch may be tough at first, especially if you find yourself sitting a lot during the day. Challenge yourself with this stretch, and remember to go slow. Your hips will thank you!

Benefits

* Loosens multiple hip muscles at once, including the gluteus medius and gluteus minimus, tensor fasciae latae, piriformis, hip abductors, hip adductors, and hip flexors.
* Improves external and internal hip rotation.
* Undoes tightness from long hours in front of a desk.
* Helps you warm up before exercise (when done dynamically).
* Helps you cool down and recover after workouts (when done statically).

Steps:

1. Sit on the floor. Bend your knees to place your heels on the floor in front of you, about double shoulder-width apart. Clasp your hands in front of your chest.
2. Keeping your chest tall, rotate your hips to one side. Lower the outside of your lead thigh and the inside of your other thigh as far toward the floor as is comfortable. Your chest should point directly over your lead knee.
3. Pause, then rotate in the opposite direction until your chest points directly over your other knee.

To Deepen This Stretch...

* Press your hands onto the tops of your knees to gently move them closer to the floor.
* Once you've rotated to the side, lower your torso over your lead knee.
* Lie flat on your back throughout the entire stretch.

Seated Figure 4

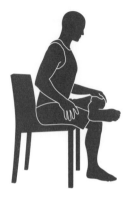

This static stretch focuses on your external hip rotators, including your piriformis. This stretch is a fundamental physical therapy treatment for relieving tension through your hip muscles. When holding this stretch, you should feel a deep stretch in the outside of your raised leg's hip. If you don't, try making micro-adjustments to your form—see the following "To Deepen This Stretch..." section—until you feel the stretch where you need it most.

Benefits
* Relieves tension through external hip rotators in the outer hip, including the glutes and the piriformis.
* Lengthens the piriformis muscle to reduce tightness, spasms, and muscle pain.
* Eases sciatic nerve irritation to reduce pain, tingling, and numbness down the hips and thighs.
* Eases lower-back pain.

Steps:

1. Sit tall in a chair with your feet flat on the floor. Cross one ankle over the opposite knee.
2. Use your hand to gently press your raised thigh toward the floor. Lean forward.
3. Hold, then switch sides.

To Deepen This Stretch...

* Lean your torso forward in small increments.
* Turn your torso to the side of your raised knee.
* Try the stretch lying faceup on the floor. Raise your planted leg from the floor and pull it toward your chest.

Hip Crossover

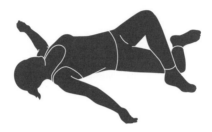

A deep figure-4 progression, the Hip Crossover deserves its own spotlight. While it lengthens your outer hips' external rotators, including your glutes and piriformis, the stretch also relieves tension in your core's obliques. This stretch helps you open up a greater available range of motion through your hips and lower back.

Benefits

* Relieves tension through external hip rotators in the outer hip, including the glutes, tensor fasciae latae, and piriformis, as well as the obliques.
* Lengthens the piriformis muscle to reduce tightness, spasms, and muscle pain.
* Eases sciatic nerve irritation to reduce pain, tingling, and numbness down the hips and thighs.
* Eases lower-back pain.

Steps:

1. Lie faceup with your knees bent and feet flat on the floor. Let your arms rest at your sides. Cross one ankle over the opposite knee.

2. Squeeze your glutes to move your raised knee away from you so that your shin runs straight across your body.
3. Rotate your torso through your hips to lower your planted leg and raised leg's foot to the floor.
4. Hold. Repeat all steps, rotating in and out of the position. Then switch sides.

To Deepen This Stretch...
* Hold the stretch for more time.
* Step the foot of your crossed-over leg closer to your opposite side's armpit.
* Gently press your raised knee away from you.

Pigeon

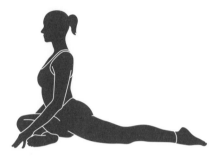

An intense yoga-inspired stretch, this pose stretches your outer, inner, and front hip muscles. In the leg that's bent, expect a deep stretch through your external rotators, including your piriformis and groin. In the leg that's stretched, your hip flexors get their own lengthening.

Benefits
* Relieves tension through external hip rotators, groin, and hip flexors.
* Lengthens the piriformis muscle to reduce tightness, spasms, and muscle pain.
* Eases sciatic nerve irritation to reduce pain, tingling, and numbness down the hips and thighs.
* Reduces excess forward pull of the hip flexors on the pelvis.
* Eases lower-back pain.

Steps:
1. Get on your hands and knees with your hands under your shoulders and your knees under your hips.
2. Bend one knee to the floor directly in front of you.

3. Slide the opposite leg behind you with the top of your foot flat on the floor.
4. Square your hips and even out your body weight between both sides of your body.
5. Hold, then switch sides.

To Deepen This Stretch...
   * Position your front shin perpendicular with your body.
   * Slowly walk your hands out in front of you. Lower your head and chest to the floor.

Standing Hip-Flexor Stretch

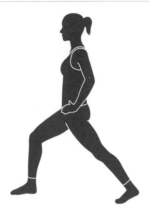

Throughout the day, get up from your desk, couch, or chair and try this stretch. It simultaneously gets you up on your feet, warms up your thigh and leg muscles, and elongates your (likely tight) hip flexors. While maintaining the position for thirty seconds or longer will give the deepest stretch possible, mixing up your holds with dynamic flows in and out of the position boosts blood flow through your thighs and glutes. This stretch can even get your heart pumping and improve your balance.

Benefits
* Relieves tension through the hip flexors.
* Reduces excess forward pull of the hip flexors on the pelvis.
* Eases lower-back pain.
* Strengthens the gluteus maximus, the largest muscle in the human body, and the quads.
* Trains balance and stability.
* Improves form during lower-body exercises by warming up the hips and legs.

Steps:

1. Stand with your feet hip-width apart, then step one leg back to come into a wide split-stance position. Raise the heel of your back leg off the floor.
2. Bend your front knee to lower your torso a few inches.
3. Squeeze your glutes to lock and square your hips. (You should not have an arch in your lower back.)

To Deepen This Stretch...

* Lower farther, or until your front thigh is parallel with the floor.
* Slowly raise and lower a few inches, without bouncing.
* As you hold the bottom position of the stretch, slowly twist your torso to face one side, then the other.
* Raise the hand on your back leg's side and gently bend in the opposite direction while reaching overhead.
* Raise both arms straight overhead.

Kneeling Hip-Flexor Stretch

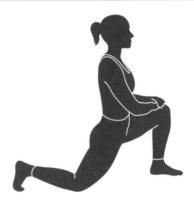

By lengthening your hip flexors from a kneeling position, this static stretch works your quadriceps in the front of your thighs. The stretch also reduces any workload on your glutes or thighs to support your body. When you really need to relieve hip flexor or quadricep tightness, this stretch is for you.

Benefits
* Relieves tension through the hip flexors and quadriceps in the front of the thighs.
* Reduces excess forward pull of the hip flexors on the pelvis.
* Eases lower-back pain.
* Trains balance and stability.

Steps:
1. Get into a kneeling position on the floor. Extend one leg behind you with a bent knee and your toes pointed toward the floor. (Place your back knee on a cushion if you need to.)
2. Squeeze the glutes of your back leg to lock and square your hips. (You should not have an arch in your lower back.)

To Deepen This Stretch...
   * Grab your back foot with the same side's hand and gently pull it toward your glutes.
   * Facing away from the front of a couch or chair, rest the top of your back foot on the edge of the seat.
   * As you hold the stretch, slowly twist your torso from side to side.
   * Raise the hand on your back leg's side and gently bend in the opposite direction while reaching overhead.
   * Raise both arms straight overhead.

Side Squat

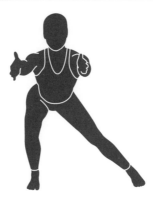

The Side Squat stretches the hip adductors (inner thigh muscles) of one leg while strengthening the abductors (outer hip muscles) of the other. For the greatest benefit—as well as to reduce any excess stress on the knee—follow these form pointers: Take a very wide stance so that your bent knee is directly over your ankle, and sit back rather than straight down, so that your weight is centered in your heels.

Benefits
* Relieves tension through the hip flexors and quadriceps in the front of the thighs.
* Reduces excess forward pull of the hip flexors on the pelvis.
* Eases lower-back pain.
* Trains balance and stability.

Steps:
1. Stand with your feet about double shoulder-width apart and your arms straight in front of you for balance.
2. Push your hips back behind you and bend one knee to lower to that side as far as possible.

3. Pause, then press through your bent leg's heel to stand back up.
4. Repeat or alternate sides.

To Deepen This Stretch...

* Hold for more time.
* Take a wider stance and lower yourself farther into the stretch—so that your leg bends as far as it can comfortably go. Let your straight leg's toes raise off of the floor.

Side-Kneeling Inner-Thigh Stretch

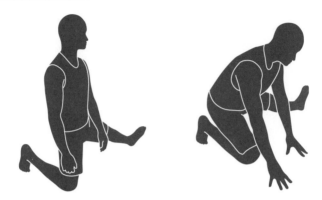

You'll feel a dynamic hip stretch in your hip adductors, the inner thigh muscles that extend from your pelvis and attach to your femur, or thigh bone. This stretch warms up both your hip flexors and hip extensors (think glutes). When doing this stretch before a workout, prioritize moving gently. If the stretch feels too intense, limit how far you lower your hips with each rep.

Benefits
- * Relieves tension through the hip adductors.
- * Improves the hips' ability to abduct, or move the legs out to the sides.
- * Warms up the hip flexors and extensors.
- * Trains balance and stability.

Steps:
1. Get on your knees with a tall torso and straight back. Extend one leg out to the side and place your foot flat on the floor.

2. Push your hips back to lower them toward the heel of your bent knee's heel. Keeping your back straight, place your hands on the floor for balance.
3. Pause, then reverse the motion to straighten your hips and raise your torso.

To Deepen This Stretch...
* Lower your hips closer to your heel and your chest closer to the floor.

Frog

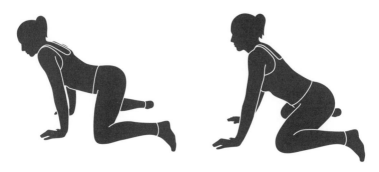

A dynamic stretch for the hip adductors, internal rotators, and groin, this stretch is a great way to loosen up before any lower-body work-out. Easing excessive tension in these muscles improves your hip alignment and stability for better leg function and helps reduce the risk of aches and pains in the hips, knees, and ankles. This stretch can get intense, so start off moving through a relatively small range of motion. As you get a sense for how your body reacts, you can think about lowering farther into the stretch.

Benefits
* Relieves tension through the hip adductors, internal rotators, and groin.
* Improves the hips' ability to abduct, or move the legs out to the sides.
* Improves the hips' ability to externally rotate, or spread the knees apart.
* Gives a gentle stretch to the lower back.

Steps:

1. Get on the floor on your hands and knees and spread your knees apart as far as is comfortable. Let the insides of your feet rest on the floor.
2. Keeping your hands in place and your arms straight, lower your hips back toward the floor in between your heels. Maintain a flat back.
3. Hold, then raise your hips and shift your weight forward.

To Deepen This Stretch...

*   Hold it statically.
*   Lower farther, or all of the way, to the floor.
*   Spread your knees farther apart.

Happy Baby

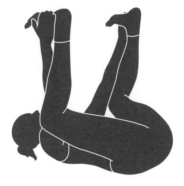

Lull yourself into deep relaxation with this lying-down yoga-inspired stretch. Providing a strong yet gentle opening to your inner hips, it requires minimal "work" (just a gentle pull through your arms). Try it at the end of workouts, before bed, or whenever you need some hip-tension relief. Breathe in deeply through your nose and out through your mouth, inflating and deflating your abdomen to give your gut and lower back a gentle stretch.

Benefits
* Relieves tension through the hip adductors, internal rotators, and groin.
* Improves the hips' ability to abduct, or move the legs out to the sides.
* Improves the hips' ability to externally rotate, or spread the knees apart.
* Gives a gentle stretch to the lower back.
* Calms the mind and body.

Steps:

1. Lie faceup and tuck your tailbone to press your lower back into the floor.
2. Bend your knees into your chest, then spread them out to your sides. Grab each foot from its outside edge with your arms outstretched.
3. Use your arms to gently widen your legs and pull your knees toward your chest.

To Deepen This Stretch...

* Gently rock from side to side, massaging your lower back on the floor.

Roll to Crawl

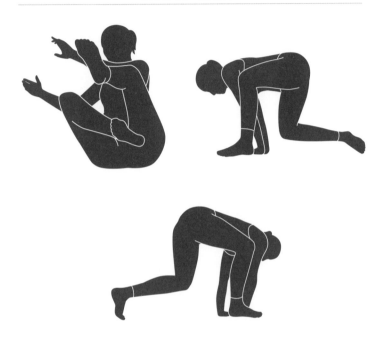

A gentle and dynamic stretch, Roll to Crawl requires (and builds) mobility in your hips, knees, and ankles. Try this stretch throughout the day or before exercise to get the blood flowing. When doing the stretch to warm up, pay attention to any muscles or joints that feel tight or restricted. Also notice any different sensations between your left and right sides. These muscles might need some extra attention.

Benefits

* Relieves tension through the internal and external rotators as well as the calves.
* Warms up the entire lower body as well as the core and shoulders.
* Increases blood flow throughout the entire body.
* Promotes mobility through the hips, knees, and ankles.
* Improves form during lower-body exercises.

Steps:

1. Sit on the floor with your knees bent and feet flat on the floor.
2. Rotate your body to one side, crossing the opposite side's leg in front of you and placing that foot flat on the floor.
3. Continue the rotation to place both hands on the floor near your opposite foot.
4. Shift your body weight into your arms and raise up onto the ball of your trailing foot.
5. Immediately rotate to the opposite side and switch legs.

To Deepen This Stretch...

* Press more through your planted foot and hands to raise your hips higher toward the ceiling.

Deep-Squat Rock

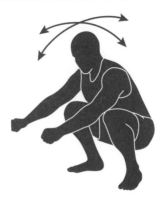

This squat is not about strength; it's all about hanging out in the bottom position, letting your bones and joints prop you up, and gently moving your body weight to open up your hips and ankles. To make the stretch easier, you can spread your feet wider. If you experience any knee pain, substitute this dynamic stretch with another one like Happy Baby.

Benefits

* * Relieves tension through the glutes and calves.
* * Warms up the entire lower body as well as the core.
* * Increases blood flow throughout the lower body.
* * Promotes mobility through the hips and ankles.
* * Improves form during lower-body exercises.

Steps:

1. Stand with your feet about shoulder-width apart and extend your arms in front of you for balance. You can also hold on to a chair or sturdy piece of furniture if needed.

2. Push your hips back and bend your knees to lower your hips toward the floor until your hamstrings touch your shins. Relax all your muscles to "hang" in the position.
3. While maintaining this squat position, gently rock your body forward and backward, side to side, and then in circles.

To Deepen This Stretch...

* Narrow your stance.
* Move farther in each direction. (You may need to take a wider stance or hold on to a chair for balance.)

Standing Quad Stretch

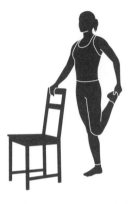

While still releasing the deeper muscles of the hips, the Standing Quad Stretch focuses on the entire length of the quadriceps from hips to knees.

Benefits

* Relieves tension through the quadriceps and hip flexors.
* Reduces excess forward pull of the quadriceps and hip flexors on the pelvis.
* Eases lower-back pain.
* Strengthens the side of the standing leg.

Steps:

1. Stand tall with your feet together, and place your hand on a wall or sturdy object for balance. Shift your weight to one leg, then bend the opposite knee to raise that foot toward your hip. Hold the top of your foot with that side's hand.
2. Gently pull your heel toward your hip. Square your hips and knees.

To Deepen This Stretch...

* Squeeze your glutes to lock your bent leg's hip.

Side-Lying Quad Stretch

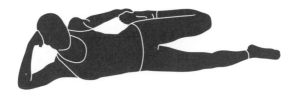

Another quad-pull stretch, this static stretch works your muscles from a side-lying position, which makes it ideal for anyone who has trouble standing on one leg or wants to simply stretch for relaxation.

Benefits

* Relieves tension through the quadriceps and hip flexors.
* Reduces excess forward pull of the quads and hip flexors on the pelvis.
* Eases lower-back pain.
* Calms the mind and body.

Steps:

1. Lie on your side with your legs straight. Support your head on your bottom side's hand.
2. Bend your top leg's knee to move your foot toward your hip. Hold the top of your foot with your top hand.
3. Gently pull your heel toward your hip. Square your hips and knees.

To Deepen This Stretch...

* Squeeze your glutes to lock your bent leg's hip.

Hip-Hinge Toe Touch

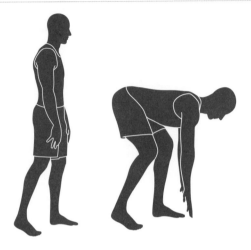

Similar to bending over and touching your toes, this stretch focuses on all the hamstring benefits without the knee pain that can occur when bending to the floor with straight legs. This stretch also works the higher portion of your hamstrings and into your glutes.

Benefits

* Relieves tension through the hamstrings and lower fibers of the glutes.
* Improves pelvic alignment and hip mobility.
* Eases lower-back pain.
* Improves form during lower-body exercises (when done dynamically).

Steps:

1. Stand with your feet hip-width apart and step one foot behind you so that your back foot's toes are in line with your front foot's heel. Raise your back heel from the floor.
2. Keeping a flat back, push your hips back behind you to lower your torso. Reach your hands to the floor, allowing a slight bend in your knees.
3. Hold, then switch sides.

To Deepen This Stretch...

* Stretch both legs at the same with your feet next to each other.
* Straighten your knees to feel the stretch in your lower, rather than upper, hamstrings.

Hamstring-Calf Switch

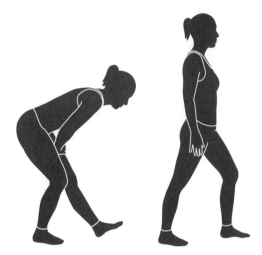

This two-for-one stretch elongates the entire back of your legs, from hips to ankles. Remember, the ankle bone is connected to the knee bone. And by stretching your muscles and joints between them, you train different parts of your body to work together. You can do this stretch statically for some in-depth muscle relaxation. However, to get the most benefit, try this stretch dynamically, flowing smoothly from one position to the other.

Benefits

* Relieves tension through the hamstrings and calves.
* Improves hip and ankle mobility.
* Eases lower-back pain.
* Improves form during lower-body exercises (when done dynamically).

Steps:

1. Stand with your feet hip-width apart and step one foot a couple of feet behind you. Raise your back heel from the floor.
2. Keeping a flat back, push your hips back behind you and straighten your front leg, raising your toes and flexing your foot toward you. You should feel a stretch in your front leg's hamstrings.
3. Leading with your chest, lower your upper torso and reach your hands toward the sides of your foot.
4. Pause, then push your hips forward and straighten your back leg, reaching your heel toward the floor. You should feel a stretch in your back leg's calf.
5. Pause, then move back into the hamstring stretch and repeat.
6. Complete the number of reps that work for you, then switch sides.

To Deepen This Stretch...

* Hold for more time.
* Spread your feet farther apart so you have more of a forward and backward lean during each phase.

Banded Ankle Distraction

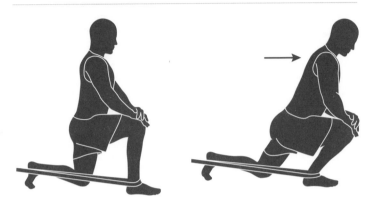

If limited ankle mobility gets in the way of your lower-body exercises like squats, this is the pre-workout stretch you need. In this stretch, looping a resistance band across the front of your ankle gently presses on—almost retracting—your foot's talus bone, giving the rest of your ankle more room to move. Try doing some body-weight squats before the Banded Ankle Distraction, and then try squats again. The second time, you may be able to lower more deeply.

Benefits

* Relieves tension through the calves, with the greatest focus on the soleus (the muscle that runs below your knee to your ankle joint).
* Improves ankle mobility.
* Trains balance and stability.
* Improves form during lower-body exercises (when done statically or dynamically).

Steps:

1. Attach a resistance band to a low, sturdy object just a few inches off the floor.
2. Facing away from the anchor point, get down on one knee with your front leg bent and your ankle directly under your knee. Loop the free end of the band around your ankle, right where your foot slopes up to connect to your shin. The band should be taut.
3. Keeping your front foot's heel on the floor, shift your weight forward so that your knee extends past your toes.
4. Hold, then repeat for all reps. Switch sides.

To Deepen This Stretch...

* Shift your body weight farther forward to try to reach your front leg's shin closer to your foot.
* Hold for more time.

Standing Plantar Fascia Pull

Even if you don't have plantar fasciitis, you'll feel the benefits of this static stretch to your foot's arch. After all, any time you're not sitting or lying down, you're on your feet, and your plantar fascia is working under the weight of your entire body. If you have heel or arch pain, try this stretch first thing in the morning before getting out of bed. You can also try this stretch when warming up for exercise.

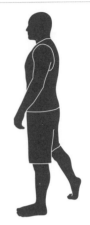

Benefits

* Relieves tension through the plantar fascia.
* Improves foot mobility.
* Eases plantar fasciitis.
* Promotes arch health and foot biomechanics.

Steps:

1. Stand with your feet hip-width apart and step one foot behind about a foot or so.
2. Raise the heel of your back foot to come up onto the ball of your foot. Allow a slight bend in your back knee.
3. Press the ball of your foot into the floor while shifting your back leg forward and your heel up toward the ceiling.

To Deepen This Stretch...

* Do the stretch facing a wall. Place your hands against the wall, one foot behind you, and then lean forward to rest your chest against the wall and further extend your back leg's foot.

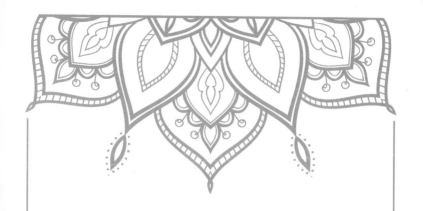

PART 3

SEQUENCES FOR EVERY STRETCHING NEED

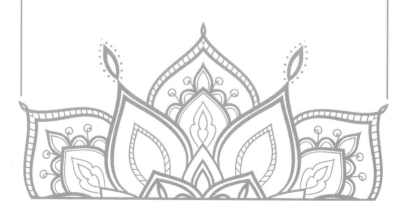

Once you are comfortable with a number of stretches, you can start putting them together into sequences—gently transitioning from one stretch to another in a natural flow of movement. In this part, you'll find stretching routines for every stretching need. From when you first wake up in the morning, to pre-workout warm-ups and post-workout cooldowns, to total-body flexibility, stretching at your desk, reducing stress, and getting better sleep, you'll find multiple stretching sequences that you can modify to fit what you're looking for.

MORNING WAKE–UP ROUTINE 1

1. **Side-Lying Quad Stretch:** Roll over in bed to lie on one side with your legs straight. Bend your top leg's knee to move your foot toward your hip. Hold the top of your foot with your top hand and gently pull your heel toward your hip. Squeeze your glutes. Hold each side for thirty seconds.

2. **Hip Crossover:** Roll onto your back and, with bent knees, cross one ankle over the opposite knee. Squeeze your glutes to move your raised knee away from you. Rotate your torso to lower your raised foot to the bed. Hold each side for thirty seconds.

3. **Pelvic Tilt:** Lying on your back, bend your knees and place your feet on the bed, hip-width apart. Squeeze your abs and tuck your tailbone to press your lower back against the bed. Hold for five seconds, then repeat for five sets.

4. **Rounded-Back Knee Pull:** Sit up on the bed with your knees bent and feet flat on the bed in front of you, shoulder-width apart. Wrap your arms around the outsides of your thighs

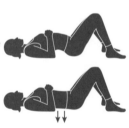

and grab your wrists under your knees. Curve your spine forward and lean back. Hold for fifteen seconds, release, and repeat for two sets.

5. **Butterfly:** Place your palms on opposite shoulders. Raise your elbows straight in front of you, then squeeze through the front of your shoulders and chest and pull through your arms to stack your elbows. Hold for thirty seconds.

6. **Seated Twist:** Sitting tall on your bed with your legs crossed, place one hand behind you and one on the opposite knee. Gently twist your torso toward your back hand. Keep a tall, upright spine. Hold each side for fifteen seconds, then repeat for two sets.

7. **Seated Figure 4:** Sit tall on the edge of your bed with your feet flat on the floor. Cross one ankle over the opposite knee. Use your hand to gently press down on your raised thigh and lean forward. Hold each side for thirty seconds, then repeat for two sets.

8. **Joint-by-Joint Finger Flexion and Extension:** Make two tight fists, then slowly extend and spread your fingers as far as possible, moving slowly joint by joint. Reverse back into fists, and repeat for five sets.

MORNING WAKE-UP ROUTINE 2

1. **Pelvic Tilt:** While lying in bed, roll onto your back, bend your knees, and place your feet on the bed, hip-width apart. Squeeze your abs and tuck your tailbone to press your lower back against the bed. Hold for five seconds, then repeat for five sets.

2. **Overhead Curl:** Lying faceup, extend your arms and legs so your body forms one long, straight line. Squeeze your core muscles and press your lower back into the bed. Keeping your shoulders down and away from your ears, slowly curl your torso up and forward as high as is comfortable or until it and your arms are vertical, stretched high toward the ceiling. Slowly reverse the curl to lower to the bed. Do five reps.

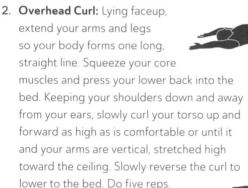

3. **Seated Side Bend:** Sit tall at the edge of the bed, raise one arm overhead, and lean toward the opposite side, keeping your other hand on the bed for support. Repeat with the other arm. Hold each side for thirty seconds.

4. **Seated Figure 4:** Sit tall on the edge of the bed with both feet on the floor. Cross one ankle over the opposite knee. Use your hand to gently press down on your raised thigh and lean forward. Hold each side for thirty seconds.

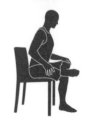

5. **Cross-Body Shoulder Stretch:** Extend one arm across your chest, keeping your elbow straight. Wrap your other arm under it and use your hand to gently pull your extended arm toward your chest. Squeeze your stretched arm's shoulder blade back and down to keep it from rounding forward. Hold each side for fifteen seconds, then repeat for two sets.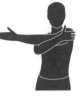

6. **Standing Reach:** Stand up with your feet together hip-width apart, and reach your arms up overhead as high as possible. Keep your shoulders down and away from your ears and avoid arching your back. Hold for thirty seconds.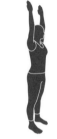

7. **Standing Hip-Flexor Stretch:** Step one leg back to come into a wide split-stance position with your front knee bent and back heel raised. Squeeze your glutes to lock and square your hips. Slowly lower a few inches toward the floor, then come back up, without bouncing. Do five reps per side. Repeat as a hold, slowly rotating your torso to face one side, then the other. Do five reps per side.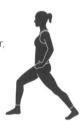

8. **Standing Quad Stretch:** Stand tall with your feet together, and place your hand on something sturdy for balance. Shift your weight to one leg, then bend the opposite knee to raise that foot toward your hip. Hold the top of your foot with that side's hand and gently pull it toward your hip. Squeeze your glutes and square both hips. Hold each side for thirty seconds.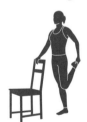

9. **Hamstring-Calf Switch:** Stand with one leg a couple of feet in front of the other and raise your back heel. Push your hips back to bend your back leg and straighten your front leg, raising your toes toward the ceiling. Pause for fifteen seconds, then move your hips forward to bend your front leg and straighten your back leg, keeping your heel on the floor. Pause for fifteen seconds. Repeat for two reps, then switch sides.

MORNING WAKE-UP ROUTINE 3

1. **Standing Reach:** Stand with your feet hip-width apart, and reach your arms up overhead as high as possible. Keep your shoulders down and away from your ears and avoid arching your back. Hold for thirty seconds.
2. **Standing Lat Dive:** Stand in front of a chair back or counter and place your outstretched arms on its edge. Push your hips back behind you to lower your torso forward until it's parallel with the floor. Hold for thirty seconds.
3. **Wrist Flexion and Extension:** Extend one arm straight in front of your shoulder with your palm facing down. Gently pull on the back of your hand. Flip your palm up, then gently pull on the palm of your hand. Hold each position for fifteen seconds, then switch sides.
4. **Reverse Shoulder Raise:** Interlace your fingers behind your back with your arms against the back of your hips. Keeping a tall torso, raise your arms toward the ceiling behind you. For a deeper stretch, rotate your wrists to face your palms away from you. Hold for fifteen seconds, release, then repeat for two sets.

5. **Hip-Hinge Toe Touch:** Step one foot just behind the other, then raise your back heel from the floor. Keeping a flat back, push your hips back to lower your torso. Reach your hands to the floor, and keep your knees slightly bent. Hold each side for thirty seconds.

6. **Standing Quad Stretch:** Stand tall with your feet together, and place your hand on something sturdy for balance. Shift your weight to one leg, then bend the opposite knee to raise that foot toward your hip. Hold the top of your foot with that side's hand and gently pull it toward your hip. Squeeze your glutes and square both hips. Hold each side for thirty seconds.

7. **Standing Plantar Fascia Pull:** Move your feet closer together and come up on the ball of your back foot. Press into the base of your toes and raise your foot until it's vertical. Hold each side for thirty seconds.

8. **Side Squat:** Stand with your feet double shoulder-width apart and your arms straight in front of you. Bend one knee, and push your hips back to that side. Hold each side for fifteen seconds, then repeat for two sets.

PRE-WORKOUT WARM-UP 1

1. **Band Pull-Apart:** Stand tall and hold a resistance band at both ends in front of your chest. Keeping your arms straight, stretch the band to your sides using only your shoulders. Slowly reverse to the front. Repeat for ten reps.

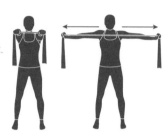

2. **Shoulder Rotation:** Lower the band in front of your thighs. Using only your shoulders and without arching your back, move the band up and behind your hips. Reverse to the front. Repeat for ten reps.

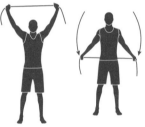

3. **Wall Slide:** Stand against a wall with your arms out to your sides like goalposts. Keeping your hips back, with shoulders and arms as close to the wall as possible, extend your arms overhead. Then slowly lower down. Repeat for ten reps.

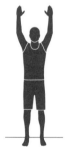

4. **Cat-Cow:** Get on your hands and knees with your knees under your hips and your wrists under your shoulders. Exhaling, slowly tuck your tailbone and drop your chin to round your back toward the ceiling. Inhaling, slowly tilt your tailbone and chin toward the ceiling to drop your back toward the floor. Repeat for five reps.

5. **T-Spine Extension:** Kneel in front of a chair or couch and place your bent elbows on its edge with your palms facing you. Hold a band or dowel. Lower your head and torso toward the floor. Hold for five seconds, release, and repeat for five sets.

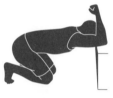

6. **T-Spine Rotation:** Get on your hands and knees and place one hand behind your head. Slowly rotate through your torso to drop your elbow toward the floor, then up toward the ceiling. Do five reps, then switch sides.

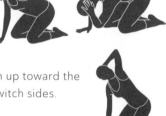

7. **Figure 8:** Relax your arms to your sides. Make relaxed fists with both hands, palms facing down. Rotate your wrists in a figure 8 or infinity shape. Do ten reps, then repeat in the opposite direction.

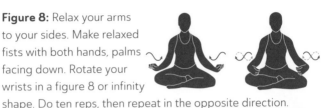

8. **Wrist Flexion and Extension:** Extend one arm straight in front of your shoulder with your palm facing down. Gently pull on the back of your hand for one second. Flip your palm up, then gently pull on the palm of your hand for one second. Do five reps, then switch sides.

9. **Wrist Flexion with Finger Touch:** Get on your hands and knees and place the backs of your hands on the floor with your fingers pointed toward your body. Touch your thumbs to each of your four fingers. Do five reps.

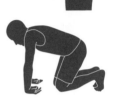

PRE-WORKOUT WARM-UP 2

1. **Banded Ankle Distraction:** Attach a resistance band to a low, sturdy object. Get on one knee, bend your front leg, and loop the free end of the band around your front ankle. Lean forward against 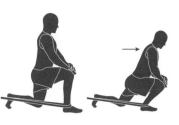 the band to lower your shin toward your foot. Pause for ten seconds, then release. Do five reps, then switch sides.

2. **Hamstring-Calf Switch:** Stand with one leg a couple of feet in front of the other and raise your back heel. Push your hips back to bend your back leg and straighten your front leg, raising your toes toward the ceiling. Pause for two seconds, then move your hips forward to bend your front leg and straighten your back 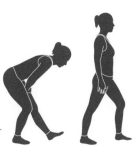 leg, keeping your heel on the floor. Pause for two seconds. Repeat for five reps, then switch sides.

3. **Deep-Squat Rock:** Stand with your feet shoulder-width apart and lower your hips all the way to the floor. Resting in this position, rock forward, backward, side to side, and in circles. Repeat for thirty seconds.

4. **Side-Kneeling Inner-Thigh Stretch:** Lower onto your knees, then extend one leg straight out to your side, foot flat on the floor. Slowly push your hips behind you to lower your torso, and place your hands on the floor. Pause for two seconds, then squeeze your glutes to raise your torso. Do five reps, then switch sides.

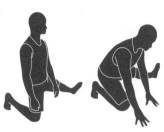

5. **90-90:** Sit on the floor with both legs bent in front of you and heels on the floor. Clasp your hands in front of your chest. Rotate your torso to one side, then the other, letting your legs fall to the floor in the direction you move. Hold each position for five seconds. Do five reps.

6. **Hip Crossover:** Lower your back to the floor and, with bent knees, cross one ankle over the opposite knee. Squeeze your glutes to move your raised knee away from you. Rotate your torso to lower your raised foot to the floor. Pause for two seconds, then squeeze through your core to raise back up. Repeat for five reps, then switch sides.

7. **Glute Bridge:** Bend your knees and place your feet on the floor near your hips. Tighten your abs to brace your core, then press through your heels and squeeze your glutes to raise your hips. Pause for two seconds, then slowly lower. Do ten reps.

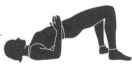

8. **Standing Hip-Flexor Stretch:** Stand with your feet hip-width apart, then step one leg back to come into a wide split-stance position with your front knee bent and back heel raised. Squeeze your glutes to lock and square your hips. Slowly lower a few inches toward the floor, then come back up, without bouncing. Do five reps per side. Repeat as a hold, slowly rotating your torso to face one side, then the other. Do five reps per side.

9. **Side Squat:** Stand with your feet double shoulder-width apart and your arms straight in front of you. Bend one knee, and push your hips back to lower to that side. Hold each side for three seconds, then repeat for ten sets.

PRE-WORKOUT WARM-UP 3

1. **Cat-Cow:** Get on your hands and knees with your knees under your hips and your wrists under your shoulders. Exhaling, slowly tuck your tailbone and drop your chin to round your back toward the ceiling. Inhaling, slowly tilt your tailbone and chin toward the ceiling to drop your back toward the floor. Repeat for five reps.

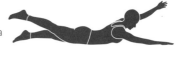

2. **Contralateral Limb Raise:** Lie facedown with your arms and legs extended in a straight line. Squeeze your glutes and upper back to raise one leg and the opposite arm a few inches from the floor. Pause for one second, then lower your arm and leg and switch sides. Do five reps.

3. **T-Spine Rotation:** Get on your hands and knees and place one hand behind your head. Slowly rotate through your torso to drop your elbow toward the floor, then up toward the ceiling. Do five reps, then switch sides.

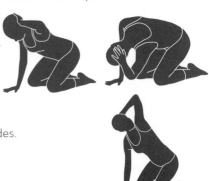

4. **Seated Side Bend:** Sit up tall, raise one arm overhead, and lean toward the opposite side, keeping your other hand on the floor for support. Hold each side for five seconds, then repeat for three sets.

5. **Serratus Roll:** Stand up and press a foam roller against a wall in front of you using the sides of your hands. Pull your shoulders forward, then slowly roll the roller up and down the wall by straightening and bending your arms. Do ten reps.

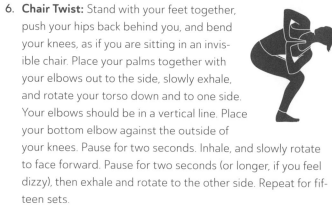

6. **Chair Twist:** Stand with your feet together, push your hips back behind you, and bend your knees, as if you are sitting in an invisible chair. Place your palms together with your elbows out to the side, slowly exhale, and rotate your torso down and to one side. Your elbows should be in a vertical line. Place your bottom elbow against the outside of your knees. Pause for two seconds. Inhale, and slowly rotate to face forward. Pause for two seconds (or longer, if you feel dizzy), then exhale and rotate to the other side. Repeat for fifteen sets.

7. **Pelvic Tilt:** Lying on your back, bend your knees and place your feet on the floor, hip-width apart. Squeeze your abs and tuck your tailbone to press your lower back against the floor. Hold for five seconds, then repeat for five sets.

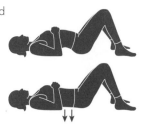

8. **Overhead Curl:** Extend your arms and legs against the floor so your body forms one long, straight line. Press your lower back into the floor and slowly curl your torso up and forward until you're sitting straight up and your arms are vertical, stretched high toward the ceiling. Slowly reverse the curl to lower to the floor. Do ten reps.

POST-WORKOUT COOLDOWN 1

1. **Overhead Triceps:** Raise one arm overhead and bend that elbow, dropping the forearm between your shoulder blades. With your other hand, gently press your elbow toward your ear and your arm down your back. Hold each side for thirty seconds.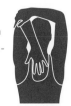

2. **Cross-Body Shoulder Stretch:** Extend one arm across your chest, keeping your elbow straight. Wrap your other arm under it and use your hand to gently pull your extended arm toward your chest. Squeeze your stretched arm's shoulder blade back and down to keep it from rounding forward. Hold each side for thirty seconds.

3. **Doorway Pec:** Stand in the middle of a doorway, place your palms on both sides, and step forward a couple of feet with one foot. Straighten your arms. Lean forward to deepen the stretch. Hold for thirty seconds.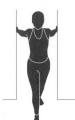

4. **Seated Biceps:** Sit on the floor with your knees bent and arms extended straight behind you, shoulder-width apart, fingers pointing away from you. Slide your hips forward and away from

your hands. Hold for thirty seconds.

5. **Thread-the-Needle:** Get on your hands and knees, then turn one hand and slide it palm-up across the floor past your opposite shoulder. Rotate your torso and lower your upper back and head against the floor. Hold each side for thirty seconds.

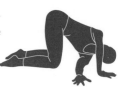

6. **Standing Lat Dive:** Stand in front of a chair back or counter and place your outstretched arms on its edge. Push your hips back behind you to lower your torso forward until it's parallel with the floor. Hold for thirty seconds.

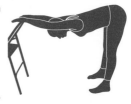

7. **Rounded-Back Knee Pull:** Sit on the floor with your knees bent and feet flat on the floor in front of you. Wrap your arms around the outsides of your thighs and grab your wrists under your knees. Curve your spine forward and lean back. Hold for fifteen seconds, release, and repeat for two sets.

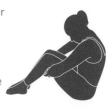

8. **Chin-to-Chest Pull:** Interlace your fingers behind your head, then gently pull your chin toward your chest. Point your elbows forward and let your upper back round. Hold for fifteen seconds, release, and repeat for two sets.

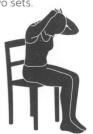

POST-WORKOUT COOLDOWN 2

1. **Standing Reach:** Stand with your feet hip-width apart, and reach your arms up overhead as high as possible. Keep your shoulders down and away from your ears and avoid arching your back. Hold for thirty seconds.

2. **Standing Lat Dive:** Stand in front of a chair back or counter and place your outstretched arms on its edge. Push your hips back behind you to lower your torso until it's parallel with the floor. Hold for thirty seconds.

3. **Seated Twist:** Sitting tall on the floor with your legs crossed, place one hand behind you and one on the opposite knee. Gently twist your torso toward your back hand. Keep a tall, upright spine. Hold each side for thirty seconds.

4. **Seated Side Bend:** From a seated position, raise one arm overhead and lean toward the opposite side, keeping your other hand on the floor for support. Repeat with the other arm. Hold each side for thirty seconds.

5. **Thread-the-Needle:** Get on your hands and knees, then turn one hand and slide it palm-up across the floor past your opposite shoulder. Rotate your torso and lower your upper back and head against the floor. Hold each side for thirty seconds.

6. **Cat-Cow:** Slide your knees under your hips and your wrists under your shoulders. Exhaling, slowly tuck your tailbone and drop your chin to round your back toward the ceiling. Inhaling, slowly tilt your tailbone and chin toward the ceiling to drop your back toward the floor. Repeat for five reps.

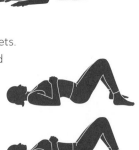

7. **Sphinx:** Lying facedown, extend your legs behind you on the floor. Support your upper body on your forearms, elbows under your shoulders. Press your forearms, pelvis, and tops of your feet against the floor to raise your head toward the ceiling. Hold for fifteen seconds, release, then repeat for two sets.

8. **Pelvic Tilt:** Lying on your back, bend your knees and place your feet on the floor, hip-width apart. Squeeze your abs and tuck your tailbone to press your lower back against the floor. Hold for five seconds, then repeat for five sets.

POST-WORKOUT COOLDOWN 3

1. **Standing Reach:** Stand with your feet hip-width apart, and reach your arms up overhead as high as possible. Keep your shoulders down and away from your ears and avoid arching your back. Hold for thirty seconds.

2. **Chair Twist:** Stand with your feet together, push your hips back behind you, and bend your knees as if you are sitting in an invisible chair. Place your palms together with your elbows out to the side, slowly exhale, and rotate your torso down and to one side. Your elbows should be in a vertical line. Place your bottom elbow against the outside of your knees. Pause for fifteen seconds. Inhale, and slowly rotate to face forward. Exhale and rotate to the other side. Repeat for two sets.

3. **Cross-Body Shoulder Stretch:** Extend one arm across your chest, keeping your elbow straight. Wrap your other arm under it and use your hand to gently pull your extended arm toward your chest. Squeeze your stretched arm's shoulder blade back and down to keep it from rounding forward. Hold each side for thirty seconds.

4. **Doorway Pec:** Stand in the middle of a doorway, place your palms on both sides, and step forward a couple of feet with one foot. Straighten your arms. Lean forward to deepen the stretch. Hold for thirty seconds.

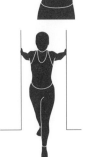

5. **Standing Quad Stretch:** Stand tall with your feet together, and place your hand on something sturdy for balance. Shift your weight to one leg, then bend the opposite knee to raise that foot toward your hip. Hold the top of your foot with that side's hand and gently pull it toward your hip. Squeeze your glutes and square both hips. Hold each side for thirty seconds.

6. **Hamstring-Calf Switch:** Stand with one leg a couple of feet in front of the other and raise your back heel. Push your hips back to bend your back leg and straighten your front leg, raising your toes toward the ceiling. Pause for fifteen seconds, then move your hips forward to bend your front leg and straighten your back leg, keeping your heel on the floor. Pause for fifteen seconds. Repeat for two reps, then switch sides.

7. **Side Squat:** Stand with your feet double shoulder-width apart and your arms straight in front of you. Bend one knee, and push your hips back to lower to that side. Hold each side for fifteen seconds, then repeat for two sets.

8. **Frog:** Get on your hands and knees, and spread your knees apart as far as is comfortable. Let the

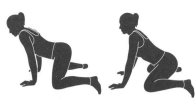

insides of your feet rest on the floor. Keeping your hands in place, lower your hips back toward the floor in between your heels, with a flat back. Hold for thirty seconds.

9. **Child's Pose:** Narrow your knees to just farther than hip-width apart with your hands under your shoulders. Keeping your hands in place, lower your hips to the floor in between your heels and bend your torso forward to the floor. Rest your forehead onto the floor. Hold for thirty seconds.

TOTAL-BODY FLEXIBILITY ROUTINE 1

1. **Shoulder Rotation:** Hold one end of a resistance band in each hand, with your hands roughly double shoulder-width apart and your arms extended in front of your thighs. Using only your shoulders and without arching your back, move the band up and behind your hips. Reverse to the front. Repeat for fifteen reps.

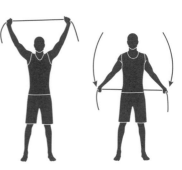

2. **Figure 8:** With your arms at your sides, make relaxed fists with both hands, palms facing down. Rotate your wrists in a figure 8 or infinity shape. Do ten reps, then repeat in the opposite direction.

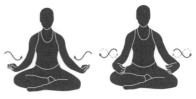

3. **Wall Slide:** Stand against a wall with your arms out to your sides like goalposts. Keeping your hips back, shoulders and arms as close to the wall as possible, extend your arms overhead. Then slowly lower down. Repeat for ten reps. Do two sets.

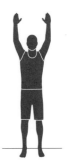

4. **Standing Hip-Flexor Stretch:** Stand with your feet hip-width apart, then step one leg back to come into a wide split-stance position with your front knee bent and back heel raised. Squeeze your glutes to lock and square your hips. Slowly lower a few inches toward the floor, then come back up, without bouncing. Do five reps per side. Repeat as a hold, slowly rotating your torso to face one side, then the other. Do five reps per side. Do two sets.

5. **Hamstring-Calf Switch:** From the same split-stance, push your hips back to bend your back leg and straighten your front leg, raising your toes toward the ceiling. Pause for two seconds, then move your hips forward to bend your front leg and straighten your back leg, keeping your heel on the floor. Pause for two seconds. Repeat for five reps, then switch sides. Do two sets.

6. **Seated Twist:** Sitting tall on the floor with your legs crossed, place one hand behind you and one on the opposite knee. Gently twist your torso to face your back hand. Keep a tall, upright spine. Hold each side for thirty seconds, then repeat for two sets.

7. **90-90:** Bend both legs in front of you and place your heels on the floor. Clasp your hands in front of your chest. Rotate your torso to one side, then the other, letting your legs fall to the floor in the direction you move. Hold each position for ten seconds. Do five reps.

8. **Pelvic Tilt:** Lower your back onto the floor with your knees bent and feet flat on the floor, hip-width apart. Squeeze your abs and tuck your tailbone to press your lower back against the floor. Hold for five seconds, then repeat for ten sets.

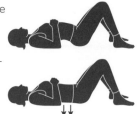

TOTAL–BODY FLEXIBILITY ROUTINE 2

1. **Kneeling Hip-Flexor Stretch:** Place one knee on the floor and extend the other leg behind you, toes pointed toward the floor. Squeeze your glutes to lock your back hip. Lean slightly forward. For a deeper stretch, grasp the top of your back foot with that side's hand. Hold each side for thirty seconds. Do two sets.

2. **T-Spine Extension:** Kneel in front of a chair or couch and place your bent elbows on the edge with your palms facing you. Hold a band or dowel. Lower your head and torso toward the floor. Hold for thirty seconds, release, and repeat for two sets.

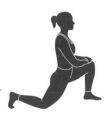

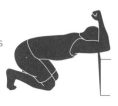

3. **T-Spine Rotation:** Get on your hands and knees and place one hand behind your head. Slowly rotate through your torso to drop your elbow toward the floor, then up toward the ceiling. Do five reps, then switch sides.

4. **Behind-the-Back Lock:** Sit cross-legged and raise your torso. Raise one arm and place that hand on your upper back. Wrap your other arm behind you and place the back of your hand on your lower back. Reach both hands toward each other, with your top elbow pointing to the ceiling, and your bottom elbow toward the floor. Hold for five seconds, release, and repeat for five sets. Switch sides.

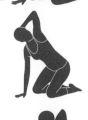

5. **Frog:** Get on your hands and knees, and spread your knees apart as far as is comfortable. Let the insides of your feet rest on the floor. Keeping your hands in place, lower your hips back toward the floor in between your heels, with a flat back. Hold for thirty seconds.

6. **Pigeon:** Bend one leg in front of you on the floor. Slide your other leg behind you, foot flat on the floor. For a deeper stretch, lower your chest to the floor. Hold each side for thirty seconds.

7. **Supine Spinal Twist:** Roll onto your back with your knees bent and feet flat on the floor. Relax your arms straight out to your sides with your palms facing up. Drop your knees to one side until they reach the floor. Turn your head and upper back to face the opposite side of your body. Try to keep both shoulder blades flat against the floor. Hold each side for thirty seconds. Repeat for three sets.

TOTAL-BODY FLEXIBILITY ROUTINE 3

1. **Contralateral Limb Raise:** Lie 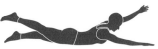 facedown with your arms and legs extended in a straight line. Squeeze your glutes and upper back to raise one leg and the opposite arm a few inches from the floor. Pause for one second, then lower your arm and leg and switch sides. Do five reps.

2. **Glute Bridge:** Roll onto your back 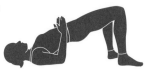 with your knees bent and feet on the floor near your hips. Squeeze your abs to brace your core, then press through your heels and squeeze your glutes to raise your hips. Pause for two seconds, then slowly lower. Do two sets of twenty reps.

3. **Banded Ankle Distraction:** 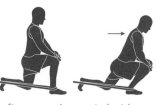 Attach a resistance band to a low, sturdy object. Get on one knee, bend your front leg, and loop the free end of the band around your front ankle. Pause for ten seconds, then release. Do five reps, then switch sides.

4. **Side Squat:** Stand up with your feet double 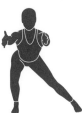 shoulder-width apart and your arms straight in front of you. Bend one knee, and push your hips back to lower to that side. Hold each side for thirty seconds, then repeat for two sets.

5. **Chair Twist:** Bring your feet together, push your hips back behind you, and bend your knees as if you are sitting in an invisible chair. Place your palms together with your elbows out to the side, slowly exhale, and rotate your torso down and to one side. Your elbows should be in a vertical line. Place your bottom elbow against the outside of your knees. Pause for fifteen seconds. Inhale, and slowly rotate to face forward. Pause for fifteen seconds (or longer, if you feel dizzy), then exhale and rotate to the other side. Repeat for two sets.

6. **Band Pull-Apart:** Hold a resistance band at both ends in front of your chest. Keeping your arms straight, stretch the band to your sides using only your shoulders. Slowly reverse to the front. Repeat for ten reps. Do two sets.

7. **Shoulder Rotation:** Hold the band in front of your thighs. Using only your shoulders and without arching your back, raise the band up and behind your hips. Reverse to the front. Repeat for ten reps. Do two sets.

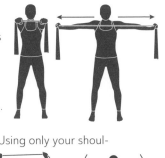

AT-YOUR-DESK RELAXER 1

1. **Segmented Chin Square:**
   Seated at your desk, relax your
   arms to your sides, then slowly
   draw a square in the air with
   your chin, pausing for five seconds at each corner. Do three
   reps, then switch directions.

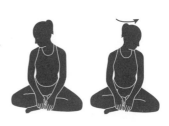

2. **Ear-to-Shoulder:** Place one hand on the opposite side of your head, above your ear. Gently and slowly pull your head to draw your
   ear toward that side's shoulder, keeping your
   shoulders down and relaxed. Hold each side
   for fifteen seconds, then repeat for two sets.

3. **Chin-to-Chest Pull:** Interlace your fingers
   behind your head, then gently pull your chin
   toward your chest. Point your elbows forward
   and let your upper back round. Hold for ten
   seconds, release, and repeat for three sets.

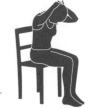

4. **Active Shoulder Roll:** Relax your arms to your
   sides, then squeeze your shoulder, chest, and
   upper-back muscles to
   raise then slowly roll your
   shoulders in a large circle.
   Do five reps, then switch
   directions.

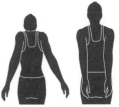

5. **Butterfly:** Place your palms on opposite shoulders. Raise your elbows, then squeeze through your chest and pull through your arms to stack your elbows. Hold for five seconds, then repeat for five reps.

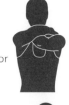

6. **Cross-Body Shoulder Stretch:** Extend one arm across your chest, keeping your elbow straight. Wrap your other arm under it and use your hand to gently pull your extended arm toward your chest. Squeeze your stretched arm's shoulder blade back and down to keep it from rounding forward. Hold each side for fifteen seconds, then repeat for two sets.

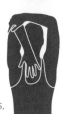

7. **Overhead Triceps:** Raise one arm overhead and bend that elbow, dropping the forearm between your shoulder blades. With your other hand, gently press your elbow toward your ear and your arm down your back. Hold each side for fifteen seconds, then repeat for two sets.

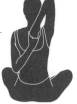

8. **Behind-the-Back Lock:** Keeping one arm raised and your hand on your upper back, wrap your other arm behind you and place the back of your hand on your lower back. Reach both hands toward each other, with your top elbow pointing to the ceiling, and your bottom elbow toward the floor. Hold for five seconds, release, and repeat for five sets. Switch sides.

AT-YOUR-DESK RELAXER 2

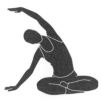

1. **Seated Side Bend:** From a seated position, raise one arm overhead and lean toward the opposite side, keeping your other hand on the chair for support. Hold each side for fifteen seconds, then repeat for two sets.

2. **Figure 8:** Drop your arms to your sides. Make relaxed fists with both hands, palms facing down. Rotate your wrists in a figure 8 or infinity shape. Do ten reps, then repeat in the opposite direction.

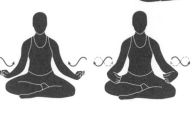

3. **Wrist Flexion and Extension:** Extend one arm straight in front of your shoulder with your palm facing down. Gently pull on the back of your hand. Flip your palm up, then gently pull on the palm of your hand. Hold each position for fifteen seconds, then switch sides. Do three sets.

4. **Standing Hip-Flexor Stretch:** Stand with your feet hip-width apart, then step one leg back to come into a wide split-stance position with your front knee bent and back heel raised. Squeeze your glutes to lock and square your hips. Slowly lower a few inches toward the floor, then come back up, without bouncing. Do three reps per side. Repeat as a hold, slowly

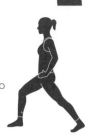

rotating your torso to face one side, then the other. Do three reps per side.

5. **Kneeling Hip-Flexor Stretch:** Lower onto one knee and extend the other leg behind you, toes pointed toward the floor. Squeeze your glutes to lock your back hip. Lean slightly forward. Grab your back foot for a deeper stretch. Hold each side for two fifteen-second holds, then repeat for two sets.

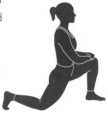

6. **Segmented Chin Square:** Sitting tall in your chair, relax your arms to your sides, then slowly draw a square in the air with your chin, pausing for five seconds at each corner. Do three reps, then switch directions.

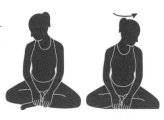

7. **Ear-to-Shoulder:** Place one hand on the opposite side of your head, above your ear. Gently and slowly pull your head to draw your ear toward that side's shoulder, keeping your shoulders down and relaxed. Hold each side for fifteen seconds, then repeat for two sets.

AT-YOUR-DESK RELAXER 3

1. **Side Squat:** Stand with your feet double shoulder-width apart and your arms straight in front of you. Bend one knee, and push your hips back to lower to that side. Hold each side for three seconds, then repeat for ten sets.

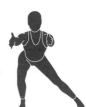

2. **Standing Quad Stretch:** Stand tall with your feet together, and place your hand on something sturdy for balance. Shift your weight to one leg, then bend the opposite knee to raise that foot toward your hip. Hold the top of your foot with that side's hand and gently pull it toward your hip. Squeeze your glutes and square both hips. Hold each side for twenty seconds, then repeat for two sets.

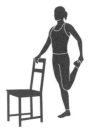

3. **Standing Hip-Flexor Stretch:** Stand with your feet hip-width apart, then step one leg back to come into a wide split-stance position with your front knee bent and back heel raised. Squeeze your glutes to lock and square your hips. Slowly lower a few inches toward the floor, then come back up, without bouncing. Hold each side for thirty seconds, then repeat for three reps.

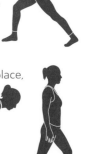

4. **Hamstring-Calf Switch:** Keeping your feet in place, take turns sitting back to straighten your front leg's hamstrings and sitting forward to straighten your back leg's calf. Pause in each position for one second. Do five reps per side, then repeat for two sets.

5. **Hip-Hinge Toe Touch:** Bring your feet a bit closer to each other, and raise your back heel from the floor. Keeping a flat back, push your hips back to lower your torso. Reach your hands to the floor, and keep your knees slightly bent. Hold each side for thirty seconds, then repeat for two reps.

6. **Reverse Shoulder Raise:** Interlace your fingers behind your back with your arms against the back of your hips. Keeping a tall torso, raise your arms toward the ceiling behind you. For a deeper stretch, rotate your wrists to face your palms away from you. Hold for ten seconds, release, then repeat for three sets.

7. **Standing Lat Dive:** Stand in front of a chair back or counter and place your outstretched arms on its edge. Push your hips back behind you to lower your torso until it's parallel with the floor. Hold for fifteen seconds, release, then repeat for three sets.

8. **I-Y-T-A:** Stand tall with your arms overhead, palms facing outward. Squeeze your shoulder blades together to slowly pull your arms back behind your shoulders a few inches. Repeat with your arms diagonally overhead, then straight to the sides, and then diagonally down and to your sides. Repeat for five sets.

9. **Doorway Pec:** Stand in the middle of a doorway, place your palms on both sides, and step forward a couple of feet with one foot. Straighten your arms. Lean forward to deepen the stretch. Hold for fifteen seconds, release, and repeat for three sets.

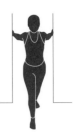

STRESS-REDUCTION FLOW 1

1. **Cross-Body Shoulder Stretch:** Sit down on the floor in a kneeling position. Extend one arm across your chest, keeping your elbow straight. Wrap your other arm under it and use your hand to gently pull your extended arm toward your chest. Squeeze your 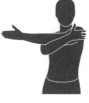 stretched arm's shoulder blade back and down to keep it from rounding forward. Hold each side for thirty seconds.

2. **Rounded-Back Knee Pull:** Bend your knees in front of you, keeping your feet flat on the floor about shoulder-width apart. Wrap your arms around the outsides of your thighs and grab your wrists under your knees. Curve 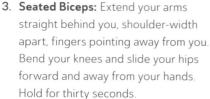 your spine forward and lean back. Hold for fifteen seconds, release, and repeat for two sets.

3. **Seated Biceps:** Extend your arms straight behind you, shoulder-width apart, fingers pointing away from you. Bend your knees and slide your hips forward and away from your hands. Hold for thirty seconds.

4. **Hip Crossover:** Lower your back to the floor and, with bent knees, cross one ankle over the opposite knee. Squeeze your glutes to move your raised knee 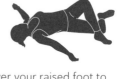 away from you. Rotate your torso to lower your raised foot to the floor. Hold each side for thirty seconds.

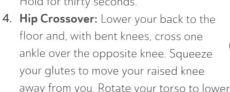

5. **Pelvic Tilt:** Lying on your back, bend your knees and place your feet on the floor, hip-width apart. Squeeze your abs and tuck your tailbone to press your lower back against the floor. Hold for five seconds, then repeat for five sets.

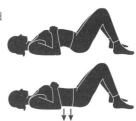

6. **Overhead Curl:** Extend your arms and legs against the floor so your body forms one long, straight line. Press your lower back into the floor and slowly curl your torso up and forward as far as is comfortable or until you're sitting straight up and your arms are vertical, stretched high toward the ceiling. Slowly reverse the curl to lower to the floor. Do two sets of five reps.

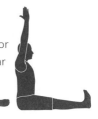

7. **Supine Spinal Twist:** Bend your knees and place your feet flat on the floor. Relax your arms straight out to your sides with your palms facing up. Drop your knees to one side until they reach the floor. Turn your head and upper back to face the opposite side of your knees. Try to keep both shoulder blades flat against the floor. Hold each side for thirty seconds.

8. **Happy Baby:** Lying flat on your back, tuck your tailbone to press your lower back into the floor. Bend your knees into your chest, grab the outsides of your feet, and drop your thighs to each side. Gently rock from side to side if desired. Hold for thirty seconds.

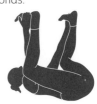

STRESS–REDUCTION FLOW 2

1. **Cat-Cow:** Get on your hands and knees with your knees under your hips and your wrists under your shoulders. Exhaling, slowly tuck your tailbone and drop your chin to round your back toward the ceiling. Inhaling, slowly tilt your tailbone and chin toward the ceiling to drop your back toward the floor. Repeat for five reps.

2. **Thread-the-Needle:** Turn one hand and slide it palm-up across the floor past your opposite shoulder. Rotate your torso and lower your upper back and head against the floor. Hold each side for thirty seconds.

3. **Side-Kneeling Inner-Thigh Stretch:** Staying on your knees, extend one leg straight out to your side, foot flat on the floor. Slowly push your hips behind you to lower your torso, and place your hands on the floor. Pause for fifteen seconds, then squeeze your glutes to raise your torso. Do two reps, then switch sides.

4. **Sphinx:** Lying facedown, extend your legs behind you on the floor. Support your upper body on your forearms, elbows under your shoulders. Press your forearms, pelvis, and tops of your feet against the floor to raise your head toward the ceiling. Hold for fifteen seconds, release, then repeat for two sets.

5. **Pigeon:** Bend one leg in front of you on the floor, keeping the other leg behind you, foot flat on the floor. For a deeper stretch, lower your chest to the floor. Hold each side for thirty seconds.

6. **Open-Hand Wrist Rotation:** From a kneeling position, place your palms on the floor with your fingers pointed toward each other and your elbows straight. Rotate your wrists a full 360 degrees until your fingers again point toward each other and your elbows face each other. Do two reps, then repeat with the backs of your hands on the floor.

7. **Frog:** Spread your knees apart as far as is comfortable. Let the insides of your feet rest on the floor. Keeping your hands in place, lower your hips back toward the floor in between your heels, with a flat back. Hold for five seconds and repeat for five reps.

8. **Child's Pose:** Narrow your knees to just farther than hip-width apart with your hands under your shoulders. Keeping your hands in place, lower your hips to the floor in between your heels and bend your torso forward to the floor. Rest your forehead onto the floor. Hold for thirty seconds.

STRESS-REDUCTION FLOW 3

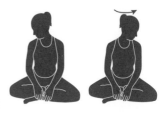

1. **Segmented Chin Square:** Sit down and relax your arms to your sides, then slowly draw a square in the air with your chin, pausing for five seconds at each corner. Do three reps, then switch directions.

2. **Ear-to-Shoulder:** Place one hand on the opposite side of your head, above your ear. Gently and slowly pull your head to draw your ear toward that side's shoulder, keeping your shoulders down and relaxed. Hold each side for thirty seconds.

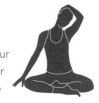

3. **Chin-to-Chest Pull:** Interlace your fingers behind your head, then gently pull your chin toward your chest. Point your elbows forward and let your upper back round. Hold for fifteen seconds, release, and repeat for two sets.

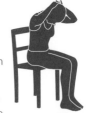

4. **Rounded-Back Knee Pull:** Sitting on the floor, bend your knees and keep your feet flat on the floor in front of you. Wrap your arms around the outsides of your thighs and grab your wrists under your knees. Curve your spine forward and lean back. Hold for fifteen seconds, release, and repeat for two sets.

5. **Seated Side Bend:** Cross your legs in front of you. Raise one arm overhead and lean toward the opposite side, keeping your other hand on the floor. Repeat with the other arm. Hold each side for thirty seconds.

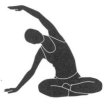

6. **Seated Twist:** Sitting tall on the floor with your legs crossed, place one hand behind you and one on the opposite knee. Gently twist your torso to face your back hand. Keep a tall, upright spine. Hold each side for thirty seconds.

7. **Overhead Triceps:** Raise one arm overhead and bend that elbow, dropping the forearm between your shoulder blades. With your other hand, gently press your elbow toward your ear and your arm down your back. Hold each side for thirty seconds.

8. **90-90:** Bend both legs in front of you and place your heels on the floor. Clasp your hands in front of your chest. Rotate your torso to one side, then the other, letting your legs fall to the floor in the direction you move. Hold each position for thirty seconds.

9. **Kneeling Hip-Flexor Stretch:** Raise onto one knee and extend the other leg behind you, toes pointed toward the floor. Squeeze your glutes to lock your back hip. Lean slightly forward. Grab your back foot for a deeper stretch. Hold each side for thirty seconds.

STRESS-REDUCTION FLOW 4

1. **Standing Reach:** Stand with your feet hip-width apart, and reach your arms up overhead as high as possible. Keep your shoulders down and away from your ears and avoid arching your back. Hold for thirty seconds.
2. **Standing Lat Dive:** Stand in front of a chair back or counter and place your outstretched arms on its edge. Push your hips back behind you to lower your torso until it's parallel with the floor. Hold for thirty seconds.
3. **Chair Twist:** Stand with your feet together, push your hips back behind you, and bend your knees as if you are sitting in an invisible chair. Place your palms together with your elbows out to the side, slowly exhale, and rotate your torso down and to one side. Your elbows should be in a vertical line. Place your bottom elbow against the outside of your knees. Pause for fifteen seconds. Inhale, and slowly rotate to face forward. Then exhale and rotate to the other side. Do two sets.
4. **Reverse Shoulder Raise:** Interlace your fingers behind your back with your arms against the back of your hips. Keeping a tall torso, raise your arms toward the ceiling behind you. For a deeper stretch, rotate your wrists to face your palms away from you. Hold for ten seconds, release, then repeat for two sets.

5. **Standing Hip-Flexor Stretch:** Stand with your feet hip-width apart, then step one leg back to come into a wide split-stance position with your front knee bent and back heel raised. Squeeze your glutes to lock and square your hips. Slowly lower a few inches toward the floor, then come back up, without bouncing. Hold each side for thirty seconds.

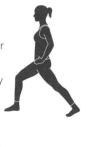

6. **Hip-Hinge Toe Touch:** Bring your feet closer together, then raise your back heel from the floor. Keeping a flat back, push your hips back to lower your torso. Reach your hands to the floor, and keep your knees slightly bent. Hold each side for thirty seconds.

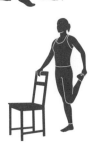

7. **Standing Quad Stretch:** Stand tall with your feet together, and place your hand on something sturdy for balance. Shift your weight to one leg, then bend the opposite knee to raise that foot toward your hip. Hold the top of your foot with that side's hand and gently pull it toward your hip. Squeeze your glutes and square both hips. Hold each side for thirty seconds.

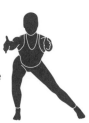

8. **Side Squat:** Stand with your feet double shoulder-width apart and your arms straight in front of you. Bend one knee, and push your hips back to lower to that side. Hold each side for fifteen seconds, then repeat for two sets.

9. **Deep-Squat Rock:** Bring your feet shoulder-width apart and lower your hips all the way toward the floor. Resting in this position, rock forward, backward, side to side, and in circles. Repeat for thirty seconds.

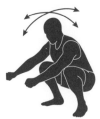

BETTER-SLEEP SEQUENCE 1

1. **Segmented Chin Square:** Sit on the edge of your bed and relax your arms to your sides. Slowly draw a square in the air with your chin, pausing for ten seconds at each corner. Switch directions.

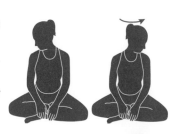

2. **Ear-to-Shoulder:** Place one hand on the opposite side of your head, above your ear. Gently and slowly pull your head to draw your ear toward that side's shoulder, keeping your shoulders down and relaxed. Hold each side for thirty seconds.

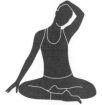

3. **Chin-to-Chest Pull:** Interlace your fingers behind your head, then gently pull your chin toward your chest. Point your elbows forward and let your upper back round. Hold for thirty seconds.

4. **Cross-Body Shoulder Stretch:** Extend one arm across your chest, keeping your elbow straight. Wrap your other arm under it and use your hand to gently pull your extended arm toward your chest. Squeeze your stretched arm's shoulder blade back and down to keep it from rounding forward. Hold each side for thirty seconds.

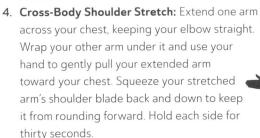

5. **Seated Side Bend:** Raise one arm overhead and lean toward the opposite side, keeping your other hand on the bed for support. Repeat with the other arm. Hold each side for thirty seconds.

6. **Thread-the-Needle:** Get on your hands and knees. Turn one hand and slide it palm-up across the bed past your opposite shoulder. Rotate your torso and lower your upper back and head against the bed. Hold each side for thirty seconds.

7. **Child's Pose:** Still on your hands and knees, keep your hands in place and your knees just farther than hip-width apart. Lower

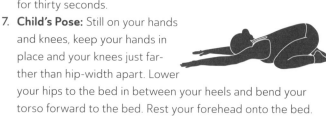

your hips to the bed in between your heels and bend your torso forward to the bed. Rest your forehead onto the bed. Hold for thirty seconds.

8. **Supine Spinal Twist:** Lie faceup on the bed, bend your knees, and place your feet flat on the bed. Relax your arms straight out to your sides with your palms facing up. Drop your knees to one side until they reach the bed. Turn your head and upper back to face the opposite side of your body. Try to keep both shoulder blades flat against the bed. Hold each side for thirty seconds.

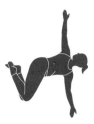

BETTER-SLEEP SEQUENCE 2

1. **Cat-Cow:** Get on your hands and knees on your bed. Make sure your knees are under your hips and your wrists are under your shoulders. Exhaling, slowly tuck your tailbone and drop your chin to round your back toward the ceiling. Inhaling, slowly tilt your tailbone and chin toward the ceiling to drop your back toward the bed. Repeat for five reps.

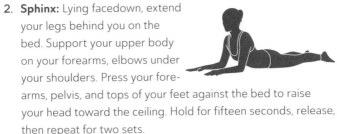

2. **Sphinx:** Lying facedown, extend your legs behind you on the bed. Support your upper body on your forearms, elbows under your shoulders. Press your forearms, pelvis, and tops of your feet against the bed to raise your head toward the ceiling. Hold for fifteen seconds, release, then repeat for two sets.

3. **Pigeon:** Bend one leg in front of you on the bed, keeping the other leg behind you, foot flat against the bed. For a deeper stretch, lower your chest to the bed. Hold each side for thirty seconds.

4. **Frog:** Come to a kneeling position, and spread your knees apart as far as is comfortable. Let the insides of your feet rest on the bed. Keeping

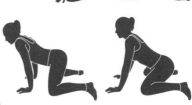

your hands in place, lower your hips back toward the bed in between your heels, with a flat back. Hold for thirty seconds.

5. **Side-Lying Quad Stretch:** Roll over onto one side with your legs straight. Bend your top leg's knee to move 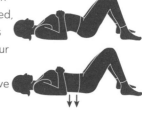 your foot toward your hip. Hold the top of your foot with your top hand and gently pull your heel toward your hip. Squeeze your glutes. Hold each side for thirty seconds.

6. **Pelvic Tilt:** Roll onto your back with your knees bent and feet on the bed, hip-width apart. Squeeze your abs and tuck your tailbone to press your lower back against the bed. Hold for five seconds, then repeat for five sets.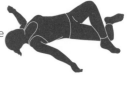

7. **Hip Crossover:** Still lying on your back, bend your knees and cross one ankle over the opposite knee. Squeeze your glutes to move your raised knee away from you. Rotate your torso to lower your raised foot to the bed. Hold each side for thirty seconds.

8. **Happy Baby:** Tuck your tailbone to press your lower back into the bed. Bend your hips and knees, grab the outsides of your feet, and drop your thighs to each side. Gently rock from side to side if desired. Hold for thirty seconds.

BETTER-SLEEP SEQUENCE 3

1. **Standing Lat Dive:** Stand in front of a chair back or counter and place your outstretched arms on its edge. Push your hips back behind you to lower your torso forward until it's parallel with the floor. Hold for thirty seconds.

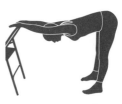

2. **Reverse Shoulder Raise:** Interlace your fingers behind your back with your arms against the back of your hips. Keeping a tall torso, raise your arms toward the ceiling behind you. For a deeper stretch, rotate your wrists to face your palms away from you. Hold for fifteen seconds, release, then repeat for two sets.

3. **Chin-to-Chest Pull:** Sit on the edge of your bed. Interlace your fingers behind your head, then gently pull your chin toward your chest. Point your elbows forward and let your upper back round. Hold for thirty seconds.

4. **Rounded-Back Knee Pull:** Scoot your lower body onto the bed. Bend your knees and keep your feet flat on the bed, about shoulder-width apart. Wrap your arms around the outsides of your thighs and grab your wrists under your knees. Curve your spine forward and lean back. Hold for thirty seconds.

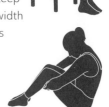

5. **Overhead Triceps:** Raise one arm overhead and bend that elbow, dropping that forearm between your shoulder blades. With your other hand, gently press your elbow toward your ear and your arm down your back. Hold each side for thirty seconds.

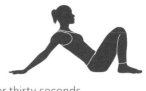

6. **Seated Biceps:** Bend your knees and extend your arms straight behind you on the bed, shoulder-width apart, fingers pointing away from you. Slide your hips forward and away from your hands. Hold for thirty seconds.

7. **Supine Spinal Twist:** Lower your back to the bed. Relax your arms straight out to your sides with your palms facing up. Drop your knees to one side until they reach the bed. Turn your head and upper back to face the opposite side of your body. Try to keep both shoulder blades flat against the bed. Hold each side for thirty seconds.

8. **Thread-the-Needle:** Get on your hands and knees. Turn one hand and slide it palm-up across the bed past your opposite shoulder. Rotate your torso and lower your upper back and head against the bed. Hold each side for thirty seconds.

9. **Child's Pose:** Still on your hands and knees, keep your hands in place and your knees just farther than hip-width apart. Lower your hips to the bed in between your heels and bend your torso forward to the bed. Rest your forehead onto the bed. Hold for thirty seconds.

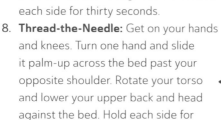

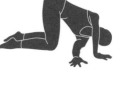

BETTER-SLEEP SEQUENCE 4

1. **Standing Hip-Flexor Stretch:** Stand with your feet hip-width apart, then step one leg back to come into a wide split-stance position with your front knee bent and back heel raised. Squeeze your glutes to lock and square your hips. Slowly lower a few inches toward the floor, then come back up, without bouncing. Hold each side for thirty seconds.

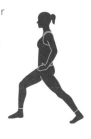

2. **Hip-Hinge Toe Touch:** Bring your feet closer together, then raise your back heel from the floor. Keeping a flat back, push your hips back to lower your torso. Reach your hands to the floor, and keep your knees slightly bent. Hold each side for thirty seconds.

3. **Side Squat:** Stand with your feet double shoulder-width apart and your arms straight in front of you. Bend one knee, and push your hips back to lower to that side. Hold each side for fifteen seconds, then repeat for two sets.

4. **Seated Figure 4:** Sit tall on the edge of your bed with both feet flat on the floor. Cross one ankle over the opposite knee. Use your hand to gently press down on your raised thigh and lean forward. Hold each side for thirty seconds.

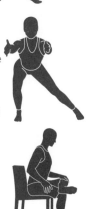

5. **Seated Twist:** Sitting tall on your bed with your legs crossed, place one hand behind you and one on the opposite knee. Gently twist your torso to face your back hand. Keep a tall, upright spine. Hold each side for fifteen seconds, then repeat for two sets.

6. **Side-Lying Quad Stretch:** Lower onto the bed and roll over onto one side. Bend your top leg's knee to move your foot toward your hip. Hold the top of your foot with your top hand and gently pull your heel toward your hip. Squeeze your glutes. Hold each side for thirty seconds.

7. **Hip Crossover:** Roll onto your back and bend your knees. Cross one ankle over the opposite knee. Squeeze your glutes to move your raised knee away from you. Rotate your torso to lower your raised foot to the bed. Hold each side for thirty seconds.

8. **Happy Baby:** Tuck your tailbone to press your lower back into the bed. Bend your hips and knees, grab the outsides of your feet, and drop your thighs to each side. Gently rock from side to side if desired. Hold for thirty seconds.

INDEX

ABOUT THE AUTHOR

K. Aleisha Fetters, CSCS, is a fitness journalist and certified strength and conditioning specialist. Currently the senior fitness editor at Livestrong.com, her work has been featured in publications including *Time*; *Women's Health*; *Runner's World*; *US News & World Report*; and *O, The Oprah Magazine*. Her books include *Give Yourself More, The Woman's Guide to Strength Training*, and *Fitness Hacks for over 50*. She is regularly interviewed as an expert for publications including *The New York Times*, *AARP*, *Lifehacker*, and *Shape*.